D1520627

GORDON M. WYANT is Professor of Anaesthesia at the University of Saskatchewan. Since 1967 he has served as leader of the Canadian delegation to the Technical Committee on Anaesthetic and Related Equipment of the International Standards Organization.

Great efforts have been made in the area of national and international standardization of anaesthetic equipment, but much remains to be done and much potentially hazardous equipment will remain in use for years to come. This book is designed to draw the user's attention to the hazards that are known to exist and to suggest how they can be minimized. It brings together published material as well as many instances that have been reported or observed.

A considerable number of these misadventures arise from inherent weaknesses in the construction of the equipment. Others result from confusing variations in the items available from different manufacturers and countries. Not only does the identification of vital parts and controls vary, but parts which should be interchangeable often or not, whereas others are described as being interchangeable when, in fact, they should never be fitted together.

The subject is discussed in a gas flow sequence, starting with the source of anaesthetic gases as they are conveyed by pipelines to the anaesthetic machine and ending at the patient's trachea.

This unique and important book should be required reading for designers, manufacturers, and maintenance personnel as well as anaesthetists.

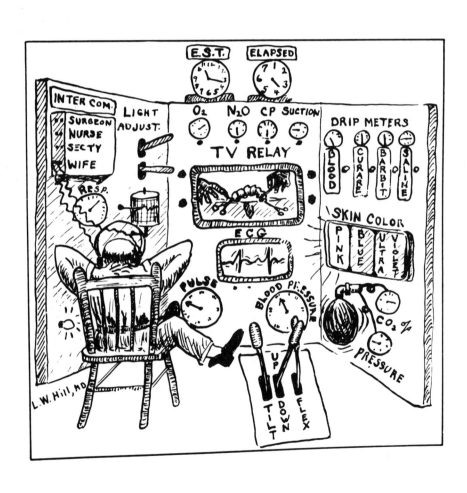

GORDON M. WYANT

Mechanical misadventures in anaesthesia

UNIVERSITY OF TORONTO PRESS
Toronto Buffalo London

© University of Toronto Press 1978
Toronto   Buffalo   London
Printed in Canada

Library of Congress Cataloging in Publication Data

Wyant, Gordon M.
    Mechanical misadventures in anaesthesia.

    Bibliography: p.
    Includes index.
    1. Anesthesiology—Apparatus and instruments—
    Accidents. I. Title. [DNLM: 1. Anesthesia—Adverse
    effects. 2. Anesthesiology—Instrumentation.
    3. Accident prevention. WO245 W974m]
    RD82.5.W93   617'.96   78-4864
    ISBN 0-8020-5423-4

To my wife, Anne

Contents

Foreword

Misadventures – or accidents – associated with anaesthesia have been studied extensively since the dawn of the specialty. The same conclusions can be drawn from these studies as from the greater number of accident investigations in all other fields of human activity: first, that few, if any, accidents can be ascribed to a single 'cause' and that numerous antecedent, contributory, and precipitating factors can always be identified; and, secondly, that many of these factors involve human failures. The latter may range from an error of judgment in a complex situation when acting under stress to the more common simple lack of care or even of courtesy. Ignorance of relevant facts often further complicates the situation.

The multifactorial aetiology of accidents is exemplified by one particular anaesthetic mishap – not involving faulty equipment – where at least thirteen people made among them twenty-five errors of omission or commission. The story is too long to unfold here, but no single one of these recorded errors would, in itself, either have 'caused' the accident or even be regarded as particularly heinous. It was their fortuitous summation that led to the fatal situation. Even so, the picture is not complete without consideration of the selection, training, and administration of the personnel involved or of the psychological or hormonal pressures to which they may have been exposed.

This involvement of the complex factors of human behaviour in the causation of accidents – and the need to present acceptable public explanation for them – readily explains why discussions on this subject arouse such strong emotions. These emotions are not confined to those who have had the misfortune to have been in an accident – or in a 'near miss' – but are shared by all those who feel that they could be involved, no matter how remotely, in a similar incident.

With accidents involving allegedly faulty equipment, this emotional response is paradoxically even more pronounced, perhaps because of our strange dichotomy of outlook towards things mechanical. On the one hand, in an age of space travel, we are conditioned to believe that machinery is, and indeed should be, infallible. On the other hand, when we see that, on earth, our motor cars, domestic machinery, and anaesthetic equipment are less than perfect, then we are unduly upset. The inanimate device which cannot answer back may often be made the scapegoat or 'cause' of the accident and provide an acceptable excuse for the errors of human behaviour. It is, after all, easier and kinder to blame the equipment and have it hastily modified than to apply the processes to the human machine.

Irrespective of these philosophical considerations, it is a fact of contemporary life that serious anaesthetic accidents, to which faulty equipment is a contributory factor, attract a degree of professional, public, legal, and even political interest which is quite disproportionate to their frequency.

It is not easy to estimate the incidence of these accidents beyond saying that it is very low for fatal ones, even though mechanical misadventures have been encountered by most practising anaesthetists. Mishaps of this kind have been reported sporadically since 1846 when it was noted that the second attempt to induce anaesthesia in London failed because of a faulty expiratory valve. This story has a contemporary flavour, as has the incident when the great Clover used a new bag which proved to have a smaller capacity than he had ordered and expected. This led to his giving a higher concentration of chloroform than intended — with, in this case, a fatal outcome. Alas, it does not appear that he tested his bag before use, though with a nominal capacity of 180 litres such a test would not have been easy! There have been many similar reports since (including the long saga to improve the Junkers chloroform inhaler) culminating in the impressive modern collection contained in this book. Instructive as all these reports are they unfortunately provide no basis for estimating the incidence of the events they describe.

More rewarding from this aspect is a study of the reviews of large series of anaesthetic deaths which have been published in the last twenty-five years. In nearly half of these no mention at all was made of any death where faulty equipment was a contributory factor, but from these series two findings are clear: first, that equipment-related deaths constituted a small percentage of the total; and, secondly, that the piece of equipment most commonly involved was simple — a tracheal tube. The situations described are well known and included obstruction by kinking or cuff herniation, oesophageal intubation, and anoxic death associated with failure to intubate.

Of the series reviewed, the largest also had by far the highest incidence (approximately 8%) of equipment related fatalities; yet in all these incidents one or more human failures could be clearly identified. It is again necessary to remember that accidents are multifactorial and it follows, therefore, that their classification is inevitably a matter of opinion varying with those factors which the compiler regards as most important.

Thus, if these human errors are felt to be of greater aetiological significance than the imperfection of the equipment, then the incidence of accidents 'caused' by faulty equipment in this series falls to 0.3% — for one incident with crossed pipelines. Some might hold the view that even the latter hazard need not necessarily lead to a patient's death, in which case the percentage of accidents 'caused' by faulty equipment would be zero.

Although this may be regarded as a harsh oversimplification since there are often extenuating circumstances, yet the study of the equipment-related deaths in these series and in other instances leads inevitably to the view that it is 'misuse' of equipment rather than its faulty design or construction which is usually the major causative factor in such accidents. 'Misuse' is used to include failure to understand the functioning and purpose of equipment, failure to check it before use and, above all, failure to recognize the clinical signs of impending disaster and to take the necessary remedial action in time. In short, 'misuse' means a failure of the anaesthetist's education.

This conclusion does not imply a denial of the importance of studying closely the small number of accidents where imperfect design or construction has played a significant role, or of the larger number where the failure has been primarily in the fields of inspection and maintenance of such equipment.

Design and construction can always be improved in the light of new knowledge and experience. Much has been achieved in other fields in designing equipment specifically to avoid or minimize hazards, accompanied by legislation to enforce safe practice, and such measures have been very effective. It is, therefore, tempting to extend these approaches to the field of anaesthesia, but it should be remembered that the problems of 'safety' in the clinical situation are seldom so neatly circumscribed as, for example, in the design of machine tools or hydraulic presses.

The overriding importance of proper education for the anaesthetist in the prevention of accidents must not be overlooked in the current enthusiasm for legislative controls for anaesthetic equipment. Some form of control is indeed desirable — particularly to minimize those hazards which are not immediately apparent to the reasonably informed user — for example, with respect to pipeline installations, electrical devices, and some equipment used chiefly in intensive care units.

It is, however, equally important that such regulations be framed so as not to impede progress and more especially to be not so all-embracing as to unduly restrict the clinical freedom of practising anaesthetists, including those who have to work with simple equipment in unsophisticated surroundings.

It is not easy to reconcile these conflicting aims – especially as there is seldom any unanimity of opinion as to when a particular hazard is sufficiently serious to merit its prescription by legislation. The opinions of anaesthetists and of engineers concerning a particular subject vary widely from: 'It could be done better'; through: 'It is a trap for the unwary'; to: 'That is downright dangerous.' Individual views are influenced by previous experience, legal decisions, established practice, and cost effectiveness. A statistical basis for decision is seldom available and the future difficult to foretell.

Moreover, in obviating one hazard it is all too easy to introduce others and a choice of evils must often be made. Several topical examples spring to mind, such as when breathing tubes are inadvertently pulled upon: should the connection to a tracheal or tracheostomy tube come apart or should it be so secure that the tube itself is pulled out? Again, should an oxygen flush valve be fitted? The need for oxygen in an emergency is undeniable, yet such devices can easily give rise to excessive pressures in the breathing system. Or, again, which is the more important – an oxygen failure alarm or a nitrous oxide cut-off device? Indeed, should the latter ever be fitted without the former, or vice versa? Should either be mandatory? Numerous other design dilemmas could be mentioned where the sometimes emotional argument always hinges around the preferred definition of 'safe practice.'

Many discussions of this kind take place on Standards Committees where, at international level, further complexities are introduced by the need to reconcile differing national, legal, fiscal, and even clinical requirements. The resulting standards inevitably arouse criticism because of their long gestation and because they, of necessity, reflect compromise. Nevertheless, the merit of a system based on voluntary agreements should not be lightly discarded in spite of its apparently leisurely working, though this may, or may not, suit the purpose of a government department subject to public pressures.

Professor Wyant is a distinguished and erudite anaesthetist who, as a respected member of the International Standards Organisation Committee on anaesthetic equipment, is well aware of these problems. He has drawn on his knowledge of the work of the committee and on his wide clinical experience in many countries to produce this unique and valuable work which contains many salutory lessons for designers, manufacturers, and maintenance personnel, as well as for anaesthetists, while re-emphasizing the classical teaching that the anaesthetist must understand and check his equipment before using it. Above all, this book will educate anaesthetists and help them to acquire that essential attribute of safe practice – a high index of informed suspicion about the vagaries of the mechanical devices which they use in their daily work.

O.P. Dinnick

MBBS (Lond), FFARCS (Eng), DA (Eng)
Senior Anaesthetist
The Middlesex Hospital
London, England

Preface

'The chapter of knowledge is very short,
but the chapter of accidents is a very long one.'

Lord Chesterfield, 1753.

The increasing complexities of anaesthetic and related equipment and the occasional malfunction with at best unpleasant and at its worst lethal effects on patients have caused us to scan the literature and review our own experiences in this regard. In doing so we have come to the conclusion that it would be useful to anaesthetists if they were able to find in one volume the common mechanical complications occurring in their trade. It has been stated, and is usually referred to as 'Murphy's Law,' that 'if a piece of mechanical apparatus can fail then it will eventually fail.' By the same token, then, whenever mechanical equipment is used anything can go wrong and one could in theory conjure up any kind of mechanical misadventure. This would be of little use to the reader and consequently the contents of this book are concerned only with those complications which have been described in the literature, have been met in personal experience, or have been communicated to us by word of mouth or from official records.

It is only fair to state that some of the information which may be found in this volume refers to complications or hazards encountered in older types of equipment and that mechanical shortcomings in many instances have been resolved by the manufacturers. Such instances have been included nevertheless, first to demonstrate what can happen even with equipment designed and produced by reputable manufacturers and secondly because some older equipment may still be in use in the unmodified original condition. Whenever modifications have been made or have been incorporated into subsequent models the author has noted it in the text wherever it has been known to him. Furthermore, since examples have been abstracted from the literature of many countries, readers may be unfamiliar with some items of equipment or with the exact manner in which they were used when the event occurred.

The subject matter under consideration can be divided essentially into three categories: (1) failure because of malfunctioning equipment; (2) failure because of interference with otherwise properly functioning equipment (wrongful re-assembly after sterilization or servicing is one example of this); (3) misuse or wrong application of functionally sound equipment. The latter, including such misadventures as insertion of a tracheal tube into the oesophagus, incorrect calculation of the concentration of volatile agents delivered by kettle vaporizers, etc. will not be covered in this volume.

In order to assist the reader in tracing malfunctions in a logical manner the subject matter is presented in gas flow sequence, starting with the oxygen source of the pipeline manifold and ending at the trachea. The subject could have been divided also on a functional basis such as sources of wrong gas administration, of hypoxic mixtures, etc., but the presentation chosen seemed to us to be the more desirable.

A number of books have been written in recent years on the subject of the functioning and mechanics of anaesthetic and related equipment* attesting to the increasing importance of and interest in this subject. This book is orientated towards malfunction and will deal with structural and functional details only insofar as knowledge in the area is necessary to the proper understanding of the text.

Any book, even one of single authorship, owes its existence to the input, direct or indirect, of many people over a considerable period of time. While it is impossible to name all those who have contributed to an author's knowledge, over and above those whose literary contributions are acknowledged in the text, there are some whose influence has been such as to leave their imprint on the entire work. It is my great pleasure to acknowledge the assistance and advice which I have received from two outstanding colleagues who have worked for many years to improve the safety of anaesthetic equipment and with whom I have had the pleasure to be associated in the field of international standardiza-tion, namely Professor L. Rendell-Baker of Mount Sinai Hospital, New York,

---

* J.A. Dorsch, and S.G. Dorsch, *Understanding anesthetic equipment: Construction, care and complications* (The Williams & Wilkins Co., Baltimore, 1975); P. Schreiber, *Anaesthesia equipment. Performance, classification and safety* (Springer-Verlag, Berlin, Heidelberg, New York, 1972); C.S. Ward, *Anaesthetic equipment. Physical principles and maintenance* (Bailliere Tyndall, London, 1975).

and Dr O.P. Dinnick of London's Middlesex Hospital. I am particularly indebted to Dr Dinnick for having graciously consented to write the Foreword to this book. Among others whose input has been invaluable and direct I should like to thank Professor R.A. Gordon of Toronto who has made valuable suggestions of an editorial nature. I count myself fortunate to have been able to enlist the co-operation of Dr D.A. Pelton of Toronto who has written the chapter on 'Pipelines,' a field in which he is an internationally acknowledged expert, and of Dr J.K. Scott of Saskatoon who has taken a special interest in the study of Scavenging Systems, and who has contributed that particular chapter. The line drawings, with the exception of Figures 2, 3, and 4, were most capably executed by Miss Jean MacGregor of the College of Medicine, University of Saskatchewan.

Many colleagues have helped me by relating personal experiences of equipment failure; their kindness is acknowledged in the text, as is that of the authors and the editors of publications who have permitted me to reproduce their illustrations. Before a manuscript is completed it goes through many stages of revision which involve repeated re-typing, a task most capably and cheerfully carried out by my secretary Mrs Kathy Kalyn, to whom I owe a great debt of gratitude for devotion to her work. Finally my thanks to the publishers, University of Toronto Press, and in particular their Science Editor, Miss L. Ourom, who has assisted in many ways and Mrs G.H. Stevenson for her painstaking copy editing.

December 1977

Gordon M. Wyant
CD, MD, FFARCS, FRCP (C)
Saskatoon

MECHANICAL MISADVENTURES IN ANAESTHESIA

I
Introduction

'The chief value in adequate physical equipment is not that it makes eternal vigilance unnecessary, but that it makes it effective.'

J.W. Horton, 1941.

An editorial in the *British Journal of Anaesthesia* of 1930 entitled 'Machines and men' (6) raised the question of a possible deterioration of clinical skills and acumen going pari passu with the development of an increasingly sophisticated technology in anaesthesia. One should remember that this was a time when the entire mechanization of anaesthesia consisted of the development of somewhat less primitive anaesthetic machines and the more common use of tracheal intubation. One wonders what the editorial writer would say today if he were to observe the practices in a modern operating room where temperature compensated vaporizers, ventilators, pulse monitors, and electrocardiographs are standard equipment, frequently joined by other complicated electronic devices. He would be pleased to see, I believe, that his dire predictions of an engineer in blue dungarees watching over a complicated instrument panel with screwdriver, oil can, and spanner outside the operating room, completely detached from the patient, have not materialized and that indeed clinical skills and the sense of responsibility towards the patient as an individual have not suffered over the years. What has changed, however, is the introduction into anaesthesia of entirely new fields of concern relating to clinical measurement, mechanics, and electronics.

It has been said that there is no need for the anaesthetist to know any more about the working of his equipment than it is for the driver of a motor car to be an engine mechanic. This analogy, however, is fallacious since the life of the patient is in immediate jeopardy if a malfunction in the anaesthetic equipment occurs, whereas in a car only tire or steering failure of all the many parts carry comparable risks for the driver. Consequently, prompt recognition of the source of failure of anaesthetic equipment and the ability to take immediate specific remedial action are imperative.

Despite the impressive improvements in the armamentarium of the anaesthetist, and bearing in mind the ever-present danger of equipment failure in even the simplest items, it behoves the anaesthetist to employ at all times the least complicated method compatible with patient safety and adequate operating conditions. The chapter on tracheal tubes might serve to underscore this tenet and to emphasize the foolishness of tracheal intubation, unless at least one of the indications for its use has been satisfied. Yet how often this simple principle is violated.

In considering the multitude of mechanical misadventures in the overall context, one must remember that those due to chemical and electrical causes are not even considered and that surely these present a group vastly more numerous and potentially as dangerous than those with which this book is concerned.

That mechanical misadventures are indeed a major problem is emphasized by the fact that reports in the literature are becoming more frequent, a fact that might be expected, given the increasing complexity of our equipment. It is interesting to note that before 1950 few reports in the literature referred to equipment failure, largely because the equipment was still relatively simple. When one then considers that the majority of cases probably never reach the journals partly for fear of litigation but largely because of sheer inertia or failure to appreciate the importance of publication as warnings against similar occurrences, it must become obvious that mechanical failures and misuse of equipment constitute a major problem in modern anaesthesia. The special committee investigating deaths under anaesthesia in New South Wales, Australia, found that 10 per cent of deaths due to anaesthesia in 1970 were due to technical mishaps (5).

As a matter of curiosity and to assure ourselves that the conditions necessary for major catastrophes did not exist in our own department, we made a quick check of our anaesthetic machines only.* To our surprise we found that all our pipeline yoke blocks, where they were used, could be inserted upside down into any yoke, thus circumventing the pin-index safety system; that on one machine the manufacturer had mislabelled the circuits (p. 21); that on two machines the Fluotec vaporizer was upstream from the Pentec (p. 52); and that while in five machines the oxygen flowmeter was upstream on the assembly, in nine others it was downstream. This situation is further complicated by the fact that the Engström ventilator has the flowmeters on the right-hand side so that downstream is on the left extremity of the assembly while in all other machines, with the flowmeter block on the left, downstream is on the extreme right. When

* These machines have now all been replaced.

checking for compliance with the international colour coding for gases (pp. 26-27), we found that two of the upstream oxygen flowmeter control knobs were white in compliance with the standard, but three were green (the non-standard US colour for oxygen), seven of the downstream oxygens were green, and on the two Engström ventilators the oxygen control knob was blue (*sic*) while the nitrous oxide one was green (p. 36), an exact reversal of the US colour usage. One can only guess at the larger national and international picture if such utter chaos can exist in one single department. A fatality has indeed occurred owing to the inadvertent closure of the oxygen flowmeter when the intention was to discontinue the flow of nitrous oxide instead, because the anaesthetist was unfamiliar with the gas sequence in a particular machine and had reached instinctively for the control knob in the position where he would usually expect to find oxygen (1).

Because of the potential hazard which such a situation represents, standards have been and are still being developed by individual countries, and more recently internationally, with the aim of arriving eventually at a point where the incidence of accidents due to mechanical failures can be greatly reduced, if not entirely eliminated. This could be achieved by making certain that non-interchangeability in some portions of the system will guarantee that the substances delivered are indeed those intended, and that (a) parts serving similar purposes are interchangeable irrespective of manufacturer, (b) flow-sensitive devices can only be attached to those portions of the breathing system in which the flow of gases is in the appropriate direction, and (c) identification of substances is uniform. That this is not an easy task, even after the appropriate standards have been agreed upon, is evident from the multitude of colour codings for medical gases, still in use many years after an international code has been accepted and published by the International Standards Organization. All standards, both national and international, are voluntary and at present few statutory provisions exist for compulsory compliance with standards. However, a trend can be discerned indicating that this may not remain so for long because both governments and the public at large are taking increasing interest in the provision of safe services and because major tragedies in the past have focused public attention on this problem. Indeed a Bureau of Medical Devices and Diagnostic Products has been established within the Food and Drug Administration of the United States of America for the purpose of setting and enforcing standards. A similar bureau exists in the Health Protection Branch of the Canadian Department of Health and Welfare.

The importance of the concept of standardization can be gleaned from the following case:

A patient who had been in a car accident and had suffered major chest injuries was transferred to our hospital. A tracheal tube had been inserted at the

*originating hospital but the connector was of non-standard dimensions having an
internal diameter of only 14 mm (Fig. 1). When the patient was received in our
Emergency Department it was impossible to ventilate the lungs either by Ambu
bag, ventilator, or by anaesthetic machine. Before adequate treatment could be
given the tracheal tube had to be changed, a procedure which involved some loss
of time and increased hypoxia.*

Yet even with equipment which fulfils all the requirements laid down by
national and international standards and which is being well maintained by
periodic maintenance, it will still be necessary to ascertain before every use that
no unforeseen leaks have developed, that vaporizers are filled and filling ports
are closed, that oxygen supply is assured – and this includes at least one full
cylinder on the machine and means for opening the valve – that all connections
fit together, and in general that the equipment is performing without faults.
Nevertheless, probably every department has incidences on file where, following
induction, the level of anaesthesia became lighter despite vaporizers being set at
increasing concentrations. There was also an inability to inflate the lungs until it
was finally determined that a filling port on a vaporizer had been left open with
the result that little of the anaesthetic agent actually reached the patient. In
other cases components may not mate one with another. While these in themselves are not mechanical failures of the equipment, they are mechanical misadventures which can be avoided by proper checking of the equipment before
use. Indeed such checks have been likened to the pilot's cockpit check, which is
a compulsory procedure before every takeoff (2, 3, 5, 7). The following example
may serve to illustrate the point:

*A 40-year-old man in ASA Physical Status VI was scheduled for drainage of a
pneumo-hydro-pyothorax. He was markedly cyanosed with tachypnoea, tachy-
cardia, hypertension, haemo-concentration, and mediastinal shift. Following
tracheal intubation and after the tracheal tube had been connected to the
anaesthetic machine, a large leak was noted in the region of the soda lime
cannister, thus making adequate ventilation of this curarized patient's lungs
impossible. Because of the precarious state of the patient and inability to identify immediately the source of the leak and thus to correct it promptly, a
second anaesthetic machine was procured, but both oxygen tanks were found
to be empty. A third machine was then obtained and ventilation was finally
carried out satisfactorily. Luckily the patient did not suffer any harm.*

None of these difficulties would have been experienced if the first machine
had been properly tested before being put into use and the life of a very sick

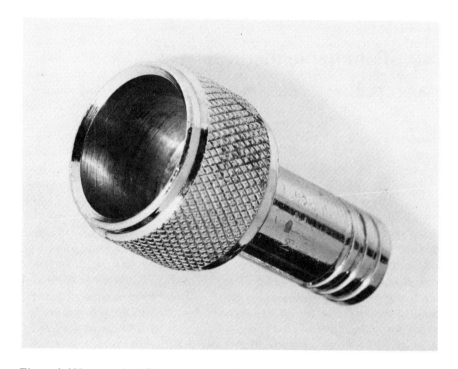

Figure 1 / Non-standard 14-mm internal diameter connector.

patient would not have been placed in considerable jeopardy. Yet, as Professor Forrester (4) pointed out in his presidential address before the Royal Society of Medicine in 1967, despite all the checks there are still some things which the anaesthetist must take on trust. One of these is that the contents of cylinders are indeed what they are purported to be and that they are free from impurities and that, where pipelines are installed, the gas issuing from a particular wall outlet is the correct one. Often errors of this nature are not recognized as early as one might expect since they may affect different practitioners and it takes some time before the apparently isolated experiences of each are co-ordinated and appraised and any mishaps traced to their source. This being so, Professor Forrester recommends the establishment in every hospital of a safety committee composed of an anaesthetist, the hospital engineer, a physicist, the fire prevention officer, and a representative or representatives from the medical staff at large and from administration. This admirable recommendation is still far from universal implementation. It is hoped that this book will prove a constructive stimulus for one aspect of the work of such a committee.

II
Non-flammable medical gas pipeline systems*

In the spring of 1973 a new addition to a large hospital in Northern Ontario was opened. On the ground floor within this new addition, medical gas pipeline systems were provided in an Emergency Treatment Room, and Out-patient Operating and Diagnostic Radiology rooms. In the next five months some hundreds of patients were treated, and in early September a young girl died during the attempted closed reduction of a supracondylar fracture of the humerus under general anaesthesia in one of the radiology rooms. This precipitated an investigation which subsequently involved another 22 deaths after the administration of medical gas in this area, and startling evidence was presented at the inquest into the 23 deaths that the oxygen and nitrous oxide pipeline systems within the new addition had been connected improperly to the pipeline systems in the existing building.

Only two general anaesthetics had been administered in this new area during the period outlined above; both ended in fatality. Nitrous oxide contributed in varying degrees to the death of the other 21 patients. They had received it from the oxygen pipelines in varying percentages through disposable face masks. Greater carnage would have occurred if the new obstetrical and surgical units on floors above had been put into use, as they were supplied with pipeline risers from the system in the new addition.

The evidence submitted at the inquest made it very clear that those responsible for designing and constructing the new addition to this hospital were totally ignorant of, or had neglected to adhere to the principles of proper and safe installation of medical gas pipeline systems, as set out in NFPA Standard 56 F (19).

* This chapter has been contributed by Dr D.A. Pelton.

Feeley and Hedley-White (9) have surveyed hospitals with anaesthesia residency programs in the United States, and among 190 replies from institutions with a central supply oxygen system and 152 which also used piped nitrous oxide there were 76 reports of malfunctions in the gas delivery systems. In 37 instances oxygen pressure was insufficient and in 6 instances pipelines had been crossed resulting in one death. There were several reports also of depletion of the nitrous oxide systems because they were too small to meet the demands.

In 1975 Wylie (25) reported that in 3 of 17 instances of equipment failure in the United Kingdom no oxygen had been delivered to the patient because of failure or mistakes in the piped oxygen supply to the operating rooms. At least one other fatal accident has resulted in the United Kingdom from a cross-connection of lines and another one in South Africa (7). Both cross-connections were made by maintenance personnel in the course of equipment modernization. In one, the terminal outlets in the wall were crossed while being refitted to the fixed pipeline; in the other new pipeline inlets with 'permanent connections to the hoses' on an anaesthetic machine-ventilator combination were concerned. In neither case were any tests carried out after completion of the work to ensure that a cross-connection had not occurred.

That pipeline failures are not all due to construction or maintenance defects but may be caused by human interference is well illustrated by the case of the workman who inadvertently drilled into the oxygen line and then turned off the supply to the operating room without notifying anyone. Fortunately no fatalities resulted from this serious transgression (7).

GENERAL CONSIDERATIONS

Medical-gas pipeline systems extend from the source of the gas to, but excluding, the anaesthetic machine and other pieces of equipment (collectively called 'terminal equipment') used in the investigation and treatment of patients. They comprise systems for oxygen, nitrous oxide, nitrogen, carbon dioxide, medical air, and medical vacuum (suction).

This chapter relates problems which have occurred in the area of medical gas pipeline systems, and presents basic safety features. It illustrates the many attributes essential to a pipeline system, so that misadventures may be avoided. The appropriate national standards should be consulted for exact details (2, 4, 6, 19). An international standard is in the course of preparation.

The ideal for maximum safety and proper functioning is being outlined. Additions and major alterations to existing systems, just as much as new facilities, should be designed and constructed in accordance with the most stringent of the national standards in force. Obviously it is not economically possible for all existing systems in all hospitals to be brought up to the ideal standard in all respects. However, safety features such as pressure regulators, relief valves, warning systems, and permanent non-interchangeable outlets and connecting assemblies are absolute minimum requirements for the protection and welfare of patients.

BASIC REQUIREMENTS OF A PIPELINE SYSTEM

A medical-gas pipeline system consists of a central supply component with control equipment, a system of pipes to the points in the facility where non-flammable medical gases may be required, and suitable station outlet valves at each point (Figs. 2A and 2B).

Source of supply
The central supply component consists of cylinders and collection equipment or of a bulk supply system which may be either permanently installed or of the trailer type. This also applies to medical air and vacuum systems. In special-care locations, such as anaesthetizing areas, recovery rooms, intensive-care and coronary-care units, an alternative source of oxygen, air, and vacuum must be readily available in case of failure of the pipeline system.

Usual hospital requirements are satisfactorily met by using a cylinder supply system with a reserve supply. Its manifold assembly should have two banks of cylinders (primary and secondary), each with its own pressure regulator and with a check valve between each cylinder and the manifold leader; the cylinders should be connected to a common header. Each bank should contain at least an average day's supply of gas. When the primary bank is exhausted, the secondary bank must function automatically to maintain supply to the pipeline. Such a cylinder system should also have a reserve supply which operates automatically in the event that both the primary and secondary systems should fail. Moreover, to prevent retrograde flow, it should have a check valve in the primary supply main, upstream of the point of connection with the secondary or reserve supply main.

An alternative to the cylinder supply is a bulk system (10, 18) which is now widely used. Such systems are being installed in new large facilities and in situations where major alterations are made to existing systems.

Medical air system
Central supply systems (Fig. 3) which supply air should comply, as a minimum, with a national standard (3). Air may be derived from a compressor system, an automatically controlled proportioning system capable of producing reconstituted air, or may come from a cylinder supply system.

A LIQUID CYLINDER SUPPLY WITH RESERVE SUPPLY

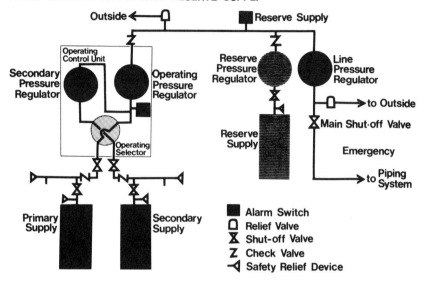

B BULK SUPPLY SYSTEM

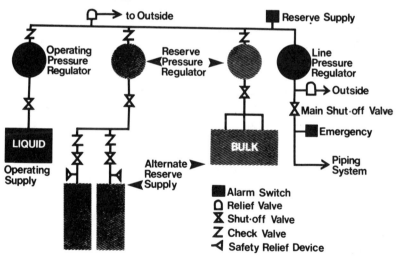

Figure 2 / Schematic drawing: A, liquid cylinder gas supply with reserve; B, bulk supply system.

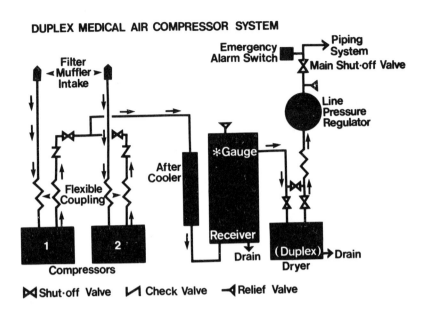

Figure 3 / Schematic drawing of a duplex medical air compressor system.

An air compressor system as a central source should consist of at least two units. Each unit must be capable of meeting the average calculated demand. It must also be fitted with an automatic alternator and controls, so that the demand will be met even if the lead unit cannot maintain an adequate supply. To satisfy these requirements, each unit must have a suitable motor starting device with overload protection, a suitable disconnect switch in the circuit, and a control circuit so arranged that shutting off one unit will not affect the operation of the other unit. The electrical system must be connected to both the regular and the emergency electrical power systems. Particular attention should be paid to the air intake component, so that the air is free of contaminants. Receivers in the system must have drains to remove condensate. Finally, the air systems must be equipped with at least two dryers to prevent water condensate accumulating in the pipelines. In special locations, because of anticipated high demand and reliance on medical air, an alternative supply of cylinder air should be available.

Medical vacuum system
A central source for vacuum (Fig. 4) must contain at least two units, each capable of satisfying average demand while the other is out of service. The

MEDICAL VACUUM SUPPLY SYSTEM

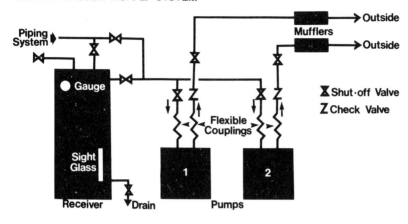

Figure 4 / Schematic drawing of a medical vacuum supply system.

system must have an automatic alternator and control to ensure that the demand on it can be met. Requirements for the electrical system, the receiver, and the exhaust are similar to those for the air compressor assembly.

General requirements for central supply systems

(1) *Cylinders and manifolds, regulators, valves, and warning systems*
Cylinders must be of proper design and construction and must be tested and maintained according to local and national regulations. Similarly, the manifolds must be of proper materials, construction, and design for the service pressures desired. Mechanical means must be provided to ensure connection to the manifold of cylinders containing the correct gas. Therefore, cylinder valve outlet connections must be of the standard for the gas involved and care must be taken to ensure non-interchangeability with other medical gases. It is generally advisable to obtain manifold assemblies from and have them installed by a manufacturer or supplier familiar with the proper practices.

There have been several reports of misadventures (16, 17, 23, 24) concerning the type of medical gases contained in cylinders and bulk reservoirs. These 'accidents' serve to underline the user's dependence upon the integrity of the manufacturer. Since it is impossible to check every item received in a hospital, these tragic happenings confirm the necessity for in-line oxygen analysers in anaesthetic machines.

Pressure regulators must be capable of maintaining a constant delivery pressure at the source at the maximal flow rate, and must be installed in the lines leading from the primary, secondary, and reserve supplies. In addition, pressure regulators capable of maintaining constant line pressure at maximal flow rate of the system must be installed in the line downstream from the changeover alarm switch and high-pressure relief valve. They must be adjustable from 50 to 60 psi (7.25 to 8.7 kPa), except for the nitrous oxide system which should be of the preset type and set at not more than 55 psi (8 kPa). The reason for recommending a preset pressure regulator for nitrous oxide is to prevent tampering with the device which might result in a higher setting and consequent higher flow, which in turn might lead to a hypoxic mixture being exhibited to the patient. This actually did occur in our hospital on two separate occasions within the span of ten days.

Each line should have a manually operated shut-off valve upstream of each high-pressure regulator, and another shut-off check valve should be installed downstream.

All pipelines, except those for nitrogen and nitrous oxide, must have a pressure-relief valve installed downstream of all pressure regulators and this valve should be set at not more than 50 per cent above the normal pressure regulator setting. The valve should relieve the pressure at a set point and be placed ahead of any shut-off valve. The nitrogen system must have a pressure relief valve, set at not more than 200 psi (29 kPa). The nitrous oxide system must have a pressure-relief valve downstream of the line pressure regulator, and this must be rated to open at 60 psi (8.7 kPa).

There are many other general factors applicable to pipeline systems, including proper location and security of the source, consideration of ambient temperature for both source and lines, and check valves in branch lines to clinical facilities and all laboratories.

All medical-gas pipelines must be equipped with pressure gauges and alarm signals for both operating and emergency systems. These should be so located as to ensure continuous visibility to responsible persons. Signals, both visual and auditory, should be installed in the office or principal working area of the person responsible for the medical-gas pipeline systems. If continuous surveillance is not assured, an auxillary visual and auditory alarm system must be provided at the telephone switchboard or other suitable location in the facility. These signal systems must be energized by both the regular and the emergency electrical power supply. Alarm systems can be divided into operating and emergency alarms.

An operating alarm system is provided on medical-gas pipeline systems that include automatic changeover from one portion of the supply to another. Both auditory and visual signals are activated when, or just before, the changeover occurs. A similar type of operating alarm system should be provided for systems in which a reserve supply is brought into service once both primary and secondary supplies are no longer functioning.

An emergency alarm system that indicates audibly and visually when the supply system is not functioning properly must be provided. This alarm system is activated by either low or high line pressures. In certain circumstances it is recommended that the emergency alarm system be activated when the reserve drops to a one-day supply. It is also recommended that a separate visual and auditory low and high pressure signal system be provided for special care locations such as anaesthetizing areas, recovery rooms, intensive care and coronary care units.

Many medical-gas pipeline systems in hospitals constructed before 1974 do not conform to existing safety standards. Faults include inadequacy of line-pressure regulators, relief valves, and warning systems (11, 21), which increase the risk of mishaps with possible fatal consequences.

(2) *Modifications to pipeline systems*

Worldwide experience in the field of modifications to existing pipeline systems in health facilities has shown the danger to be greatest when the connection is made between an altered or modified system and an existing one. A few general comments will be made concerning this type of construction, but the reader is referred for detailed information to Canadian Standards Association Standard Z305.1-1975: 'Non-Flammable Medical-Gas Piping Systems.'

To minimize the risk of cross-connection between new and existing medical-gas pipeline systems, connections to existing systems must be undertaken one at a time. The connection must not be made until pressure tests on the new addition or modification have been completed in accordance with national standards. All sections of the existing system downstream of the connection point must be taken out of service until they conform to appropriate test requirements. It is vitally important that, where an addition is made to an existing system, the new pipeline take-off must be equipped with an isolating valve at the connection point to the existing system. This isolating valve must remain in the 'off' position and be sealed throughout the installation. When the addition has been completed and the standing pressure and cross-connection tests have been completed and have been found to comply to the standard, the isolating valve should be opened to permit purging and concentration tests at the outlets of the new system.

Several fatalities have occurred after modifications to existing pipeline systems have been made, such as cross-connections in the oxygen and nitrous oxide lines, and leakage of nitrogen, used as the pressure test gas in a new oxygen line, back into the main oxygen line through a faulty valve (1, 15).

(3) *Shut-off valves and outlets*

Pipeline systems must have appropriate shut-off valves, and if they are accessible to unauthorized persons, they should be installed in valve boxes with transparent, frangible windows large enough to permit manual operating, and should be labelled appropriately. The main medical-gas supply line and each riser in the pipeline system should have shut-off valves to isolate part of the system should an emergency arise or immediate repairs be required. A manual shut-off valve should also be located convenient to a nursing station for use in an emergency.

Each station outlet for medical gas must be equipped with either a manual or an automatic shut-off valve, designed to prevent errors in cross-fitting during assembly of valves and valve bodies, clearly labelled with the name and colour code of the gas, and permanently fixed and equipped with non-interchangeable connections. If a non-interchangeable quick-coupler is used, the outlet should incorporate an automatic shut-off valve so that, when the quick-coupler is removed, the flow of medical gas will cease until the other member of the quick-coupler is reattached.

(4) *Identification of pipelines and outlets*

Modern buildings, particularly those in moderate climates, have many pipeline systems within the walls and ceilings. The pipes are copper tubing and act as conduits for various gases and liquids. In health care facilities, additional pipeline systems are installed to carry medical gases such as oxygen, nitrous oxide, medical air, and in some instances nitrogen and various gas mixtures: another pipeline system serves the need for vacuum. Unless each of these pipeline systems is properly identified, misadventures are bound to occur. This has been proven beyond doubt in the past. It is a hopeful sign that there are (or soon will be) national, or failing these, provincial or state identification markers for these different pipeline systems. Such markers must be permanent, easily identifiable, and applied to all medical-gas pipeline systems.

A suggested method of identifying these systems properly follows: all medical-gas pipelines should have permanent identifiers applied at minimum intervals of twenty feet (6 meters) before and after barriers, behind access doors, and at inlet and outlet points of each pipeline. The identifier in CSA Standard Z305.1 is a white band with red crosses and is taped to the pipeline. In addition, each separate medical-gas pipeline should be colour-coded and labelled with the name of the gas at the same place as the identifier. All labels should be self-adhesive and overlap with themselves when applied. Colour coding, in accordance with International Standards Organization Standard 32 (1975), would be advantageous (pp. 26, 27). Other countries have solved the problem in their own way by using some or all of these identifiers.

The outlets of medical-gas pipelines should have permanent identification plates, labelled as to the gas type, and preferably also colour-coded.

To minimize misadventures, it is recommended that all pipelines, fittings, manifolds, and terminal equipment be identified daily during the installation, to ensure that proper identification is maintained. In addition, the 'as-built' mechanical drawings should show only the variations of a medical-gas pipeline system from the contract drawings. Furthermore, they should be maintained on a daily basis on a separate set whenever a change is made. When construction has ended, these 'as-built' drawings must be given to the owners of the health facility for their permanent records. When alterations or additions are made, the 'as-built' drawings should be up-dated. (A tradesman working in a ceiling with a maze of copper pipes cannot ascertain absolutely the purpose of each pipe unless all are properly identified.)

(5) *Testing of pipeline systems*

During installation of a pipeline system the contractor must maintain the cleanliness of the system. When an area or section has been cleaned, it is wise to have the ends of the pipes capped. Every effort should be made to have the pipes as clean as possible before they are put into service.

Once the station outlets (terminal units) have been installed, the entire system must be subjected to pressure tests to detect leaks at joints. During these tests, particularly if it is a modification of or alteration to an existing system, the new system must in no way be connected to the existing one because the test gas used by many contractors is either dry air or nitrogen. Each separate pipeline must be back-pressured to purge it of particulate foreign matter. This obviously had not been done in a new pipeline installation for oxygen, compressed air, and nitrous oxide tested by Eichhorn and associates (8) since they found each line to contain contaminations of a volatile hydrocarbon at an initial concentration of 10 parts per million and dust of a fine gray particulate matter. These contaminants were eventually largely eliminated by purging with continuous flows of the respective gases. Specific gauges with separate non-interchangeable probes for each gas system must be employed. A common but totally unacceptable practice carried out by some installers is the use of a universal adaptor on their testing equipment.

The cross-connection test determines whether a cross-connection exists between pipeline systems for two different medical gases. The first step in this procedure is to ensure that all pipeline systems are reduced to atmospheric pressure. One system only is tested at a time, and it is pressurized with air or nitrogen. It is recommended that only air be used if the new system is an alteration or modification of an existing one. When pressurized, each station outlet is checked to determine that the test gas is being dispensed only from the outlets of the system being tested. The pressure applied to the system is 50 psi (7.25 kPa) and is measured by a gauge fitted with an adaptor specific to that system. Each system then is back-purged several times to expel the test gas.

After purging of each system, the permanent terminal outlets must be tested with a gas analyzer to confirm the presence and concentration of the appropriate gas. There are several methods available using various gas analyzers, but a relatively inexpensive, new, and reliable portable analyzer, based on gas chromatography, is manufactured by Gas Dynamics of Toronto, Canada.

The purity of each gas should be confirmed by analyzing a sample from the source and comparing it with one from the most distal outlet. A satisfactory result must show that the pipeline system has not added a contaminant to the gas under test.

Failure to test the pipeline before putting it into service has led to a number of disasters. The latest of these has befallen the Suburban General Hospital in Norristown, Pennsylvania (20).

Certification of systems

The ultimate performance test of a system, and its conformance to an acceptable and approved standard should be done by an agency experienced in this field, totally independent of contractor, gas and equipment suppliers, and the owner. If the systems fail to meet the prescribed standards, they must not be used.

Maintenance of systems

Some national standards apply only to facilities where pipeline systems are extensive and complicated. However, there are systems in small private hospitals, and in medical and dental offices, and there are no standards for these. There have been many worldwide reports of accidents (22) due to causes such as lack of gas at the source, cross-connections occurring when the pipes passed from storage rooms to terminal equipment in other rooms, and improper connections at the terminal equipment. Many of these small systems have been in existence for years and are potentially lethal because they may not have basic safety features built into their component parts. NFPA Standard 56F and CSA Standard Z305.1-1975 have sections which pay particular attention to this problem.

Connecting assemblies

The medical gas pipelines between the permanent outlets which may be located in booms, walls, floors, or ceilings and the terminal equipment have often been referred to as 'flexible hoses' or 'lines.' Some permanent fixed pipelines have flexible components as an integral part of the system, and are usually found in boom-type or ceiling units. In an attempt to avoid confusion in terminology, particularly on an international basis, the term 'connecting assemblies' will be used.

These assemblies are a matter of great concern in the fields of anaesthesia and respiratory therapy. There have been many reports of fatal accidents in Canada, the United States, Great Britain, and other countries (22).

There is at the present time no standard to prevent cross-connection of these assemblies. Misadventures have occurred because the connectors at either end have been interchangeable (16). In 1975 there were two deaths in Canada and one in Great Britain because the assemblies were crossed at the anaesthetic machine. In two the connectors were interchangeable, and in the other the connectors were torn out of the hoses, replaced, but incorrectly reattached. Two such cases have also been reported by Hunter (12), who also has pointed out that usually the connection between hoses and connectors is very secure unless tubing and connector originate from different manufacturers and so are not of exactly matching diameter (13).

National and international agencies are preparing standards for these assemblies. The important principles include: (1) the inlet and outlet connectors of the assembly must not be interchangeable, (b) the piping or tubing component must be permanently attached to them, (c) the assemblies must be repaired only by the manufacturer, and (d) the total assembly must be properly identified and labelled to conform with the appropriate standard.

SUMMARY

An attempt has been made to point out the trouble areas in medical-gas pipeline systems. Standards have been developed in many countries and the general principles on which they are based have been presented. To prevent mishaps, standards must undergo frequent review, revision, and development when necessary (5, 14). Most importantly, people must be made aware of their existence and must abide by them. In order to achieve this end it is necessary for governments to pass legislation giving standards the status of regulations under the law.

III
The anaesthetic machine

GENERAL CONSIDERATIONS

Major malfunctions of anaesthetic machines are infrequent but when they do happen they occur suddenly. Disabling malfunctions such as failures of packings and gaskets or breaking of metal or glass cannot, of course, be prevented. Schweitzer and Babarczy (10) have, for instance, found that the sealing rubber gasket on the one-way valve on the inspiratory limb on their Boyle machine was missing. This resulted in a discrepancy between the inspiratory and expiratory volumes. Ventilation was with a tidal volume of 950 ml but only 450 ml entered the expiratory limb while the remaining 450 ml was venting back into the inspiratory limb. To anticipate major malfunctions, an orderly system of regular maintenance and checks is advisable at least every three months. These checks should include oxygen failure safety valves, oxygen alarms, flow control valves, flowmeters, oxygen flush valve, delivery hose, pipeline inlet connection and hose, drawers, wheels and handles, vaporizers, pressure gauges, electrical safety and conductivity, circle system, and exclusion of leaks (3). But even such routine maintenance still does not confer an absolute guarantee against equipment failure. Hence it is imperative that before being put to use, anaesthetic equipment should undergo certain general checking procedures (p. 131). If needed, even more technical procedures are available, as described by Mayer (8).

Other misadventures may have their origin in the design or construction of the anaesthetic machine itself. For instance, some machines have separate common gas outlets for the circle and Magill breathing systems. A selector switch directs the flow of gases to one or the other outlet. In one machine the labels indicating the position of the switch for one or the other system were transposed (Fig. 5). In other models of machines the selector lever may be knocked inadvertently into the midway position, obstructing the gas flow and giving the

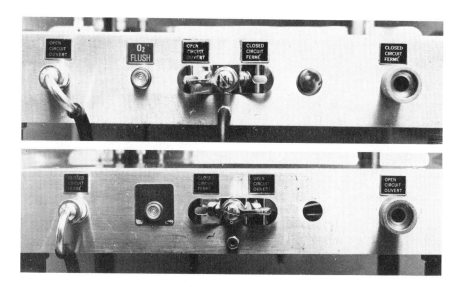

Figure 5 / Front panel of the Canadian Heidbrink Machine.
Above: incorrect labelling of outlet and valve positions.
Below: correct labelling of common gas outlets and shunt valve.

impression that both oxygen and nitrous oxide supplies have failed. Yet another example of faulty design is the Boyle Model 10 anaesthetic machine, manufactured in the United States. This machine also has two common gas outlets. The one on the upper right corner of the cabinet is the primary outlet and to it may be attached either a Magill or similar circuit or a connecting tube, as shown in Figure 6A. This connecting tube leads the gases to the absorber through a second common gas outlet located in the centre of the front of the machine (not shown). When the connecting tube is not in use, it is supposed to be placed into a storage post at the side of the machine (Fig. 6B). Longmuir and Craig (7) have had two unfortunate experiences with this machine. In both, the connecting tube had become detached from the common gas outlet, and was inserted into the storage post, with which it made an airtight seal. The resultant blockage of gas flow to the patient through the circle system caused the bag to deflate. This, together with the resultant cyanosis, led to quick recognition and correction of the situation in one case before serious harm could come to the patient. In the second case the anaesthetist activated the oxygen flush valve which is part of the Boyle Mark II absorber whenever the breathing bag needed refilling. This resulted in complete recall of the operation by the patient.

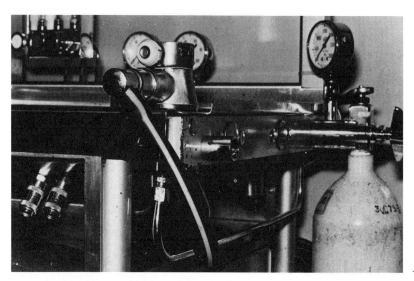

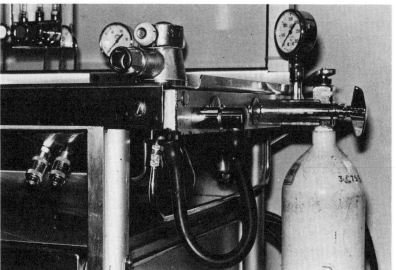

Figure 6 / Boyle Model 10 machine showing the primary common gas outlet with connecting tube
A, leading to second common gas outlet,
B, in storage position.
From Longmuir and Craig (7); courtesy: Canadian Anaesthetists' Society Journal

Dinnick (2) has pointed out recently a potential flaw in design relating to low pressure pipeline gauges which are now often found on anaesthetic machines. These gauges may be fitted on either side of the check-valve designed to prevent the escape of gas if the pipeline is not connected and cylinders are open. The precise relationship of gauge to check-valve frequently is not obvious on inspection of the machine. If the gauge is on the machine side of the check-valve, it registers not pipeline pressure, as such, but rather the pressure within the machine. If a reserve cylinder is open and the pipeline supply happens to fail, no indication of such failure will be given by the gauge until the cylinder is empty, an event which might escape notice. If, on the other hand, the gauge is on the pipeline side of the check-valve, but for one reason or another the cylinder pressure exceeds that of the pipeline, the gauge will indicate pipeline pressure while gas is drawn from the cylinder. It follows that reserve cylinders should remain closed while the pipeline is in use and flowmeters watched, whether or not a pipeline pressure gauge is fitted and what its position is in relation to the check valve.

It was customary in some older machines to have a nitrous oxide flush valve incorporated, similar to the oxygen flush. Intended to facilitate induction with nitrous oxide and still used by some for induction in children, it is a potentially dangerous fitting as it is too easy to activate the wrong flush in an emergency 12, 13). While proposed ISO standards permit the emergency oxygen control to be constructed so that it can be cocked open, it is preferable that it be of the self-closing type, otherwise there is danger that the anaesthetist may forget to close the high oxygen flow when it is no longer needed, with the result that patients are inadequately anaesthetized. The danger when the flush-valve is combined with another function, as when for instance it is made to serve as the vaporizer on/off tap, will be discussed on p. 50.

While obstruction of gas lines within the anaesthetic machine is uncommon, foreign materials such as metal shavings and chips which have not been removed after manufacture may be present and may become lodged in check valves, regulators, and needle valves (4). Austin (1) has described a relatively new machine in which loosening of the plating on the inside of the exit port was observed during routine servicing. This plating was easily rubbed off by finger pressure. X-ray examination of the rubber hoses of this machine revealed three particles of metal within the tubing, one only 5 cm from the mask. It would seem reasonable to insist that the practice of plating the inside surfaces of anaesthetic equipment be discontinued. Eger and Epstein (4) have pointed out that where flexible gas lines are used within the machine assembly they may kink or become separated and therefore should be exposed throughout their entire length to make it immediately obvious if this should occur. While this is a reasonable recommendation, most modern machines now have metal piping. However, these should be labelled at all junctions for the gas they are intended to carry. Even safer would be non-interchangeable connections.

Most machines in general use are of the constant flow variety. Intermittent flow machines, the main application of which is in obstetrics and in dentistry, are more complicated in construction. Since the working parts are largely hidden from view, it is not always possible to know with any degree of certainty whether the machine is working properly. Nainby-Luxmoore (9) has tested 50 machines, mostly of the intermittent flow variety and of almost every type and vintage. He found that the Walton-V and the A.E., a new machine resembling the Walton-V, were the only two intermittent flow machines which were free from defects and were accurate. All other Walton types, the McKesson and Jecta-flows, which is now obsolete, always had at least one representative which delivered inaccurate concentrations. Consequently it was difficult to have great confidence in any of them. The Walton-IV and II and some of the McKessons were so defective and the inaccuracies were so great or their behaviour so erratic that they constituted a real threat to patients. A similar variation in perform-ance of 85 machines of 14 different types was found by Hutchinson (6). The majority, but not all, were of the intermittent flow type. Everett, Hornbein, and Allen (5) found the McKesson Narmatic suitable for rebreathing only if the inflow was sufficiently high and spontaneous ventilation was allowed.

While oxygen, and for that matter nitrous oxide, do not explode, they speed combustion and may induce self-ignition of highly combustible material. Con-sequently, it is imperative that no greasy, oily, or other combustible lubricant be used anywhere along the high pressure portion of the gas supply. Silicone greases (Fluorolube) are often used by service men because they are non-flammable. However, they can cause foaming of the anaesthetic agent if they gain access to a bubble-through vaporizer (p. 53). Spoerel (11) cites a case in which the equip-ment orderly had used a greasy thumb to wipe off some dust from the orifice of an oxygen tank before attaching it to the anaesthetic machine. The anaesthetist who turned the tank on the following morning, thereby releasing oxygen to the reducing valve at the pressure of 180 atmospheres, was startled by a flame shooting out of the reducing valve.

COMPRESSED GAS CYLINDERS

The primary and overriding concern with cylinders must always be the identifi-cation of their contents. Bitter experience has taught that mere labelling is not sufficient to avoid errors and consequently colour and mechanical coding systems were adopted a long time ago. Subsequently, attempts were made to standardize the colour of cylinders and to extend this coding to all parts of the medical-gas system. Although consistent colour coding is not mandatory in many countries and, indeed, adherence to the internationally agreed code (ISO-32) has been spotty, significant progress has been made. A list of the international medical-gas colour codes and those in use in countries not adhering to it is given in Table I. Consequently, the ultimate guide to cylinder contents must be the label, although it is hoped that eventually the international code will be universally accepted and difficulties in identification therefore eased significantly.

Nevertheless, accidents can still occur and the user must accept on trust that the content of a cylinder is indeed that indicated by the colour coding of the cylinder, the label, or both. A number of examples are known when this was not the case. For instance one has been described (2) when cylinders for oxygen in fact contained compressed air, an error that resulted in cyanosis in four operating rooms and consequently led to analysis of the contents of the cylinders. Mazze (9) has reported the filling of oxygen cylinders with helium in order to avoid the purchase of new helium cylinders. The cylinders had not been repainted nor had the pin-index been altered. The helium label was not visible when the cylinder was hung on the anaesthetic machine. In yet another case reported in 1945 (1) a nitrous oxide cylinder was attached to the oxygen inlet of the machine, because the cylinder had been exposed to such prolonged handling and adverse weather that the colour was worn off and the label had become unreadable.

Steward and Sloan (12) report an instance in which a cylinder of helium would not fit the helium yoke but did fit the nitrous oxide pin-indexed yoke. On closer inspection it was found that the blue paint of nitrous oxide had been overpainted with the brown for helium. The valve of the cylinder revealed a deep indentation in the region opposite the No. 6 pin whereas the cylinder was pin-indexed for nitrous oxide (Nos. 3 and 5). Consequently, it would appear that the repainted cylinder had been forced onto the pin-indexed filling manifold, possibly by the use of double washers.

Not only must the identity of cylinder contents be taken on trust, but so also must their purity. This is particularly important in the case of nitrous oxide since its most common contaminant — nitric oxide — is highly toxic (3, 11).

Although a rare occurrence, oxygen cylinders have been known to explode. The most likely mechanism is a fracture compromising the integrity of the cylinder itself or of the valve, leading to the sudden escape under high pressure of the content of the cylinder which is then propelled forward like a jet-driven

TABLE I

Generally used colours for medical gas cylinders (as of October 1974)

	Air	Carbon dioxide	Carbon dioxide – oxygen	Cyclo-propane	Ethylene	Helium
ISO-32	Black-white	Gray	Gray-white	Orange	Violet	Brown
Argentina	Black-white	Gray	Gray-white	Orange	Violet	–
Australia	Black-white[2]	Gray	Gray-white[2]	Orange	Violet	Brown
Austria	Gray	Gray-black	Blue	Red-yellow	Red-yellow	Gray
Brazil	Green-black	Gray	Gray-green	Orange	Violet	Brown
Canada	Black-white	Gray	Gray-white	Orange	Violet	Brown
Colombia	Gray	Red	–	Orange	–	Red
Denmark	Black-white	Gray	Gray-white	Orange	–	Brown
Ecuador	Pink	Gray	–	Orange	–	–
Finland	Black-white	Gray	Gray-white	Orange	Violet	Brown
France	Black-white	Gray	Gray-white	Orange	Violet	Brown
Holland	Blue-green	Gray	–	Orange	Pink	Brown
Japan	Gray	Green	Gray	Gray	Gray	Gray
Mexico	Black-white	Gray	Gray-green	Orange	Red	Brown
Norway	Black-white	Gray	Gray-white	Orange	Violet	Brown
Spain	Black-white	Gray-black	Gray-white		Violet	Brown
Sweden	Black-white	Gray	Gray-white	Orange	Violet	Brown
Switzerland	Brown	Black	Black-blue	Gray	Red-gray	Yellow-green
Thailand	Green-gray	Gray	Gray-green	Orange	Red	Brown
Uruguay	Green-yellow	Gray	Gray-green	Orange	Red	Brown
U.K.	Black-white[2]	Gray	Gray-white	Orange	Violet	Brown
U.S.A.	Yellow	Gray	Gray-green	Orange	Red	Brown
Venezuela	Blue-white	Gray	Gray-green	Orange	Red	Brown
West Germany	Gray	Gray	Gray-blue	Red	Red	Gray
West Indies	White-blue	Gray	–	Orange	–	–

NOTE: Indicated colours normally apply to cylinder shoulder; balance of cylinder may be of a different colour. Dual colours shown in segments or bands visible from valve end; gray sometimes silver or aluminum.

[1] Shoulder only; body of cylinder black.
[2] Shoulder only; body of cylinder gray.
[3] Shoulder only; body of cylinder brown.
[4] Shoulder only; body of cylinder blue.
[5] Where oxygen is outside of 19.5 to 25.5% range.

Helium-oxygen	Nitrogen	Nitrogen-oxygen	Nitrous oxide	Nitrous oxide – oxygen	Oxygen
Brown-white	Black	–	Blue	–	White
–	Black	–	Blue	–	White
Brown-white[3]	Black	–	Blue	Blue-white[4]	White
Gray	Green	–	Gray-yellow	–	Blue
Brown-green	Black-gray	–	Blue	–	Green
Brown-white	Black	–	Blue	–	White
–	Brown	–	Blue	–	Green
Brown-white	Black-green	–	Blue	–	White
–	Yellow	–	Blue	–	Green
Brown-white	Black	–	Blue	–	White
Brown-white	Black	–	Blue	–	White
Brown-gray	Yellow	–	Blue-gray	–	Blue
Gray	Gray	–	Gray	–	Black
Brown-green	Black	–	Blue	–	Green
Brown-white	Black	–	Blue	–	White
Brown-white	Black	–	Blue	–	White
Brown-white	Black	–	Blue	–	White
Gray	Green	–	Green-gray	–	Blue
Green-brown	Gray	–	Blue	–	Green
Green-brown	Gray-black	–	Blue	–	Green
Brown-white	Black[2]	–	Blue	–	White
Green-brown	Black	Black-green[5]	Blue	–	Green
Brown-green	Blue-yellow	–	Blue	–	Green
Gray-blue	Green	–	Gray	–	Blue
–	Brown	–	Blue	–	Green

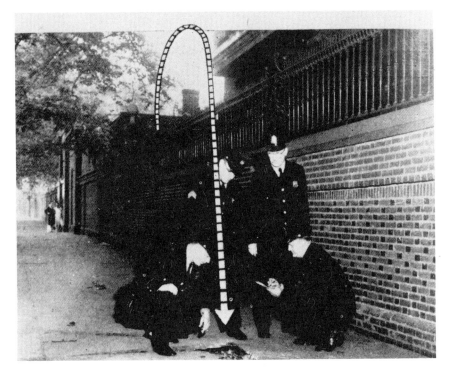

Figure 7 / Trajectory of cylinder showing site of impact on sidewalk
Courtesy: American Society of Anesthesiologists, Inc.

projectile. One such case has been described in the literature (13). In that particular case an old partial fracture, about 8 inches from the base, gradually extended around the cylinder causing it to be propelled into the air, negotiating a 10-foot high wall, and eventually landing on the sidewalk (Fig. 7). Dr. Mohelski from Vienna, who visited Cardiff about 1951, was killed when the oxygen cylinder or the reducing valve mounted on it exploded as he was opening the cylinder (10).

A similar effect may result from the inadvertent dropping of a cylinder and consequent breaking of the valve stem. A related accident has been reported by Finch (6). In this particular case, when the cylinder wrench was turned on with the intention of opening the cylinder, the entire valve stem and its retaining collar shot out of the top of the cylinder and hit the ceiling. Apparently some unidentified person, instead of using the cylinder wrench, had attempted to open the cylinder valve with a hexagonal wrench, unscrewing the valve almost completely out of the collar in the mistaken assumption that he was opening the cylinder to gas flow. With the last half-turn of the valve-seat the already loosened valve was expelled under the full pressure of the cylinder content. The suggestion is made that it would be safer if the thread direction of the valve stem were opposite to that of the valve collar, in which case 'opening' the valve collar by mistake would in actual fact tighten the thread.

Another dangerous situation can arise when the thermal safety device in the neck of the cylinder, which often is in the shape of a recessed hexagonal head, is mistaken for the normal conical depression in the valve destined to receive the retaining screw (7). This results in the high insertion of the cylinder valve into the yoke, so that the nipple cannot engage the gas exit port in the valve. Further tightening of the retaining screw will not correct the resulting leak of gases but will merely serve to drive the retaining screw deeper into the soft Wood's metal which constitutes the thermal safety device. This then may be extracted from the cylinder valve-head when the retaining screw is loosened preparatory to removal of the cylinder. If this were to happen, the contents of the cylinder would escape under great pressure and create a very hazardous situation. Rendell-Baker in discussing this situation makes the observation that the attempted wrong insertion of a cylinder in too high a position does not seem to be as rare as one might assume, to judge from evidence on cylinders which show that the thermal safety device had indeed been impinged upon in the past by a retaining screw. It would seem advisable for manufacturers to make the device in the form of a bolt rather than a recess screw head. In the United Kingdom a safety plug is not part of the cylinder valve.

Pre-mixed oxygen-nitrous oxide combinations in one cylinder in proportions of 60 to 40 per cent or 50 to 50 per cent have acquired a certain popularity. At 2000 psi (290 kPa) the critical temperature of the mixture is lowered below room temperature, permitting both gases to exist in the gaseous state with steady proportions being delivered. The use of such a mixture has been advocated as a kind of fail-safe device since obviously the loss of oxygen would entail a simultaneous loss of nitrous oxide and so be a guarantee against hypoxia due to a failing oxygen supply (5). Cooling of a 60 : 40 nitrous oxide and oxygen mixture to 0 to $-1°$ C or of a 50 : 50 mixture to $-8°$ C results in condensation of liquid nitrous oxide at the bottom of the upright cylinder (8) and this persists for one week after re-warming unless the cylinder is agitated (4), or it is immersed in water at $52°$ C and inverted three times. Failing either precaution, an oxygen rich mixture would be delivered early in the life of the cylinder with a nitrous oxide rich mixture towards the end, and this has been known to contain as little as 1.5 per cent oxygen.

PIN-INDEX SAFETY SYSTEM

The pin-index safety system was introduced in 1952, the idea having originated in the United States. It was subsequently accepted as a United Kingdom Standard (BS 1319 : 1955), as an American Standard (B57.1 : 1965), as a Canadian Standard (B96-1: 1965), and as International Standard Recommendation ISO R-407. It consists in essence of two pins as integral parts of the yoke of the anaesthetic machine. The pins are intended to mate with two corresponding holes drilled into the neck of the cylinder valve. The basic dimensions of the system are reproduced in Figure 8A, a combination of two of the six different positions being allocated to each medical gas. Thus ten different combinations are possible (Table II). In an ISO Draft Standard proposal a single hole at

TABLE II

Pin-index for compressed gas cylinders

Pin position	Cylinder content
1–3	Ethylene
1–4	Nitrogen
1–5	Air
1–6	Carbon dioxide or Carbon dioxide-Oxygen (CO_2)
2–4	Helium-oxygen (He $< 80\%$)
2–5	Oxygen
2–6	Carbon dioxide-oxygen ($CO_2 < 7\%$)
3–5	Nitrous oxide
3–6	Cyclopropane
4–6	Helium or helium-oxygen (He $> 80\%$)

position No. 7 has been assigned to a nitrous oxide-oxygen mixture of approximately equal proportions, commercially known as 'Entonox' (Fig. 8B). Consideration is now being given to twenty more sets of pin positions, which will then be available for assignment to new medical gases or mixtures (2) (Fig. 8C).

In an Editorial in the *Canadian Anaesthetists' Society Journal* (1) it has been stated that: 'Pin-indexing of gas cylinders has entirely abolished anaesthetic accidents caused by wrong positioning of cylinders on anaesthetic machines.' Unfortunately this statement is not quite true and is an expression of the false sense of security which excellent and much-needed preventive safety measures can instill into users. None of these measures can confer absolute safety. It is entirely true to say that the introduction of pin-indexing has greatly reduced the chances of wrong positioning of cylinders at the level of the anaesthetic machine, but it has by no means 'entirely abolished' such accidents as reference to the literature reveals. The seriousness of attaching a cylinder to a yoke destined

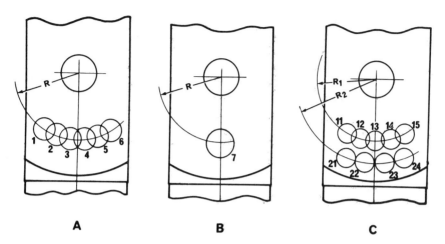

Figure 8 / A, Arrangement of pin index holes in neck of cylinder valve.
R = 14.3 mm (nominal). B, Position 7 for 'Entonox.' C, Proposal for additional
pin positions. R1 = 13.1 mm (nominal); R2 = 17.9 mm (nominal).
Courtesy: Compressed Gas Association, Inc.

for one containing a different gas was clearly recognized a long time ago, and
indeed Lundy and Seldon (6) described a method which they used at the Mayo
Clinic as early as 1941. They enlarged the strainer nipple of the oxygen yoke as
well as the port in the valve of the cylinder into which the strainer nipple is
placed. Thus oxygen could be used on any yoke, the larger port fitting the
standard nipple, but no other gas would fit the oxygen yoke since the enlarged
nipple would not mate with the smaller hole in the cylinder valve. Harroun and
Hathaway (4) described another but less reliable system used by them in 1944 to
minimize the accidental interchange of cylinders.

Eight years later in a review of 'Deaths under Anaesthetics', MacIntosh (7) still
cites three examples where cylinders had been wrongly connected by interchang-
ing oxygen and nitrous oxide, and in 1956 Edwards et al. (3) in a report of 'One
Thousand Deaths' found that one of the fatalities had been due to the attachment
to the machine of a nitrous oxide cylinder instead of one containing oxygen.

It is surprising that the implementation of the pin-index system was slow. The
British Department of Health and Social Security gave instruction in 1954 to
effect the change-over, and as most machines at that time were fitted with
'baskets' to hold cylinders rather than with yokes, the change-over was easy and
was effected relatively quickly. In the United States, on the other hand, con-
sumer indifference and even resistance to the conversion of older machines, was
a cause of occasional long delay. It is of interest to note that it was estimated as

late as 1970 that 20 to 30 per cent of hospitals in the United States did not have a pin-index safety system installed on their anaesthetic machines at that time (11) and even in 1967 Minuck (8) could still report that two fatalities in a series investigated by him were due to the administration of the wrong gas.

Yet even with pin-indexing installed, circumstances can arise in which the system fails or its provisions are circumvented. Breakage of one of the pins or forcing it into its seating hole reduces the indexing from a two-pin to a one-pin system and it can be readily seen from Table II that, if, for instance, the pin in position 2 were broken or otherwise rendered inoperative, a cylinder containing nitrous oxide or one containing air could be fitted to the yoke designed for the reception of an oxygen cylinder. While broken pins have been known to occur, few instances have been reported and the only example found in the literature is that of Wolff, Lionarons, and Mesdag (12) in which the pin indexing, rather than forming part of the yoke, was incorporated into the wall gas pipeline outlet panel. It had two nitrous oxide and two oxygen outlets, each provided with female pinholes, while the male pins were part of the coupling of the pressure tubing which led directly to the flowmeters of the anaesthetic machine. Since one pin was missing on one of the oxygen lines it could be and was connected to one of the nitrous oxide outlets, with the result that cyanosis increased whenever oxygen was flushed. The mistake was recognized before any serious harm could result, but the accident points to the need to check the identity of the gas whenever cyanosis occurs or if it increases when oxygen is being flushed. An incidental precaution might consist of having only one nitrous oxide terminal, since there is no real need for a duplicate outlet.

However, the wrong gas can be administered in the presence of an intact pin-index, since human ingenuity knows no bounds and can at times be applied to our detriment. In older anaesthetic machines with no provision for direct attachment of the piped gas supply hose to the machine, it has been customary to lead the gases into the yoke by means of a yoke block suitably provided with female pin-index holes. However, if this block is inserted upside down, an error which would, of course, never be made with a cylinder, that portion of the block which is normally above the gas outlet but now is below may be too short to impinge against the pins. Thus it becomes possible to attach a nitrous oxide or any other block to any oxygen yoke. This occurrence was first described by Rawstron and McNeil in 1962 (9) and attention was again drawn to this possibility by Steward and Sloan (10). We have a number of older machines in our department in which yoke blocks are used and we have been able to demonstrate that this inversion of the block is indeed still possible, despite the recommendation that the upper portion of blocks should be made longer to obviate this possibility (Fig. 9). Representations have been made to have the ISO Standard modified accordingly.

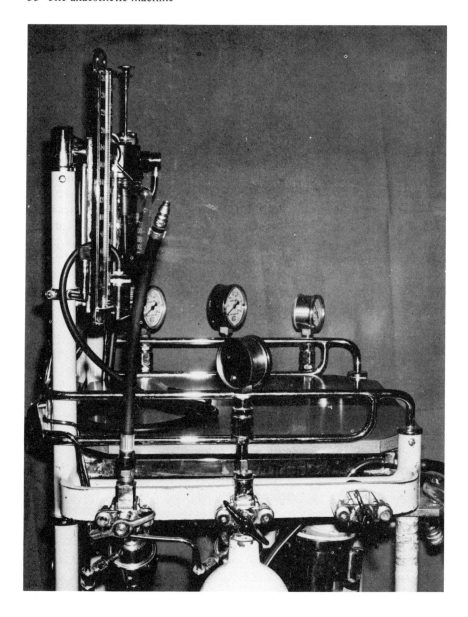

Figure 9 / Yoke block of nitrous oxide high pressure line inserted upside down into oxygen yoke, despite pin indexing.

There are still other circumstances under which the pin-index may fail. These have been described by Hogg (5). He was able to fit a nitrous oxide cylinder in a new anaesthetic machine to the cyclopropane, oxygen, and nitrous oxide yokes without detectable leakage. He also found, in an older machine, that a nitrogen cylinder had been attached to an oxygen yoke, the cylinder having been painted green, although a different shade of green than the oxygen cylinder on the other oxygen yoke. In the first case the author found that the Number 6 pin on the cyclopropane yoke had been inserted into a hole that was too deep. The depth of the hole was not specified in the Standard. When the handle was tightened, the Number 6 pin which, of course, did not mate with the Number 5 hole in the oxygen tank was simply driven deeper into the hole, thus essentially reducing the system to a one-pin system, centred on the Number 3 pin. This deficiency is being remedied in the proposed revision which requires that the design must be such that the pin protrusion cannot be reduced below the minimum by the application of force. In the second instance the interchangeability of the nitrous oxide and oxygen cylinders was due to the superimposition of two washers, one upon the other, thus reducing the effective length of the pins so that, although the cylinder was not pin-indexed, a satisfactory seal could be effected. Hogg recommends that the pin-length should be increased, that washers should be standardized, that the nipple diameter for oxygen should be different from all others (thus adding the Lundy-Seldon safeguard to the pin-index), and that colours used for medical gases should not be permitted to be used on non-medical cylinders. Specifications in the 1975 proposed revision for the pin-index deal with the first two recommendations by requiring a pin projection of 5.5 mm and a washer thickness of not more than 2.4 mm before compression. Consequently, even the use of two washers could not circumvent the protection provided by the still protruding pins.

A further example of pin-index failure, this time at the filling manifold of cylinders, has been described elsewhere in connection with an incident when a nitrous oxide cylinder was charged with helium (see p. 25).

PRESSURE REGULATORS

Relatively few instances of malfunction of pressure regulators have been described which is a tribute to the construction and sturdiness of these pressure reducing valves. Most regulators used in anaesthetic machines are of the one-stage type and are supplied to every gas on the machine, usually one for each yoke, whether this be a double or a single yoke. Cyclopropane yokes do not always have a regulator since the gas is supplied in the cylinder at relatively low pressure.

The remarkable safety record of the pressure regulator is to a large degree due to the provision of a pressure relief valve on the low pressure side. This protects the distal portions of the machine from excessive pressure should the reducing mechanism fail. Such failure of the diaphragm of the Adams-type valve has been known to occur on occasion. Hamelberg, Maffey, and Band (3) have described four incidents in which the diaphragm of nitrous oxide regulators has ruptured. The relief valve permitted the high pressure to be dissipated to the outside air. The cause of these malfunctions was traced to nitric oxide as an impurity in the nitrous oxide which had eroded the nylon diaphragm of the regulator. It might be worth mentioning at this point that failure of the diaphragm does not usually mean immediate failure of gas supply.

An incident has been described in which there was a flash and explosion as the oxygen tank was turned on, with bursting of the tubing connecting the pressure regulator to the rotameter. On inspection, the interior of the regulator was found to be melted. It seems likely that the regulator was stuck, but suddenly worked itself free, allowing oxygen to escape under high pressure into the tubing. Since the rotameter control valve was closed at the time, heat was generated by the pressure. The combination of heat and pressure in the presence of oxygen caused the rubber to burn at a rate which reached instantaneous explosive velocity. The explosion blew out the primary fire. In another case flames shot out of the reducing valve as the oxygen cylinder was turned on, but they were controlled by turning off the flow of oxygen. No damage was caused other than charring of the diaphragm of the regulator. In view of these two occurrences it is recommended that the low pressure circuit on the machine always be opened before high pressure valves are turned on (1). It is equally important to adhere to the rule that cylinders, and especially oxygen cylinders, should be opened momentarily before connecting them to the yoke to blow out any dust and that cylinder valves be opened slowly. Failure to observe these precautions has led to oxygen fires (2).

In another incident reported in the literature reducing valves were transposed during maintenance of the machine, resulting in the delivery of the wrong gas to the patient (4). While this accident is not due to malfunction of the valves themselves, it is, however, of considerable significance in view of the grave danger inherent in such gas mixups which have been alluded to several times previously. It again points to the absolute necessity of a very close check of any machine which has undergone major maintenance involving disassembly of portions of the gas conducting system.

FLOWMETERS

Flowmeters are devices designed to measure the flow of liquids or gases which are made to pass through them. In the context of the anaesthetic machine the substances to be measured are gases, usually but not invariably derived from compressed gas cylinders. The most common type of flowmeter presently in use is the rotameter, a device in which a float in the shape of a fluted bobbin is carried upwards in the lumen of a tapered tube by the gases entering from below and leaving at the top. The fluting causes the bobbin to rotate. By this definition most flowmeters installed on US machines are not true rotameters, although they bear a superficial resemblance to them. The amount of gas allowed to flow is regulated by a needle valve and the amount of flow is read from a graduated scale set behind the flowmeter tube or etched upon it. Malfunctions in a flowmeter of this kind may be due to failures of the needle valve, the flowmeter tube, or the float. On anaesthetic machines a number of such flowmeters for different gases are grouped together side by side as an integral assembly.

The needle valve and control knob
Needle valves on flowmeters serve both a control and an on-off function. Eger and Epstein (11) suggest that these two functions should be separated from one another, and this has now been done in the new Foregger 710 machine. The needle valve would then control flow so that damage from scouring of the valve seat by forceful closure would be avoided since this leads to eventual inaccuracies in gas flow control (Fig. 10).

In most machines the needle valve control knob is colour-coded, corresponding to the gas for which the particular rotameter is designed. Given the difference of colour coding for oxygen between the International Standard on the one hand and the United States, and to a lesser degree other countries, on the other hand (Fig. 11), a source for error exists, especially in view of the variable positioning of the oxygen flowmeter within the flowmeter battery (Fig. 12A, B). Aside from colour coding, it would appear desirable that the control knob for oxygen should also be distinguishable by touch, so that the machine may be used safely in a darkened operating room, or when the stress of the moment might otherwise predispose to error. One configuration for the oxygen knob has been described by Calverley (3). A draft ISO recommendation and a proposed US standard (24) provide that the oxygen flow control knob shall have a characteristic fluted profile and 'may be arranged to project beyond the knobs controlling other gases in a bank of flowmeters. Its diameter shall be not less than the diameter of knobs controlling other gases. Other flow-control knobs shall be round.' (Fig. 13) At least one manufacturer used to provide different shapes for every flowmeter control knob, but this would seem to defeat the purpose in the sense that one may not be able to remember the size and shape of the all-important oxygen flowmeter when all knobs differ from one another.

Flowmeter inaccuracies
Flowmeter inaccuracies are common and occur even in machines under continuous maintenance contracts even when they have been recently inspected and

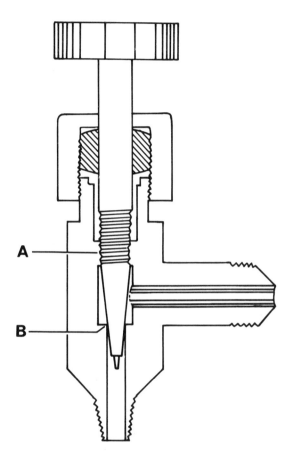

Figure 10 / Schematic cross section of a needle valve. Control over gas flow is provided by the valve thread at A and by the taper at B.
From Eger and Epstein (11); *courtesy: Anesthesiology*

maintained (28). Inaccurate measurement of flow passing through a flowmeter is one of a number of possible problems and may be due to the transposition of unmarked flowmeter tubes. This usually happens during maintenance or when a broken tube is being replaced. To prevent errors of this kind, tubes now are marked with the name of the gas for which they are designed and have an etched-on scale. Manufacturers also insist that only one tube be detached at a time. Kelley and Gable (15) describe an instance where the flowmeter from the 'Vernitrol' halothane vaporizer had been broken and replaced, including new

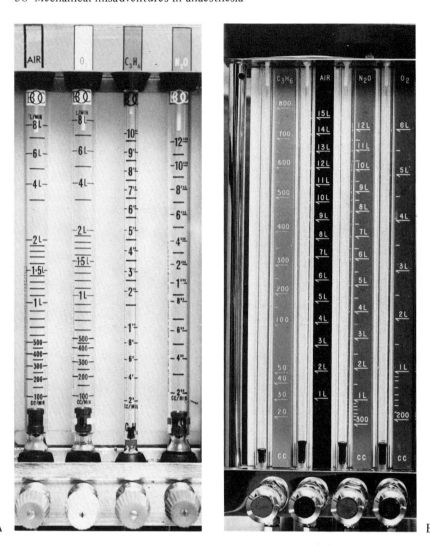

Figure 12 / A, Flowmeters of Boyle anaesthesia machine with oxygen flowmeter (white) upstream and nitrous oxide (blue) downstream. B, Flowmeters of Ohio machine with oxygen (green) downstream.

scale, tube and bobbin, by a maintenance man. When the machine was next used a strong smell of halothane was detected, certainly too strong for the intended concentration as indicated by the flowmeter. On analysis it was found that at the 250 ml/min setting of the flowmeter 1 500 ml were actually being delivered,

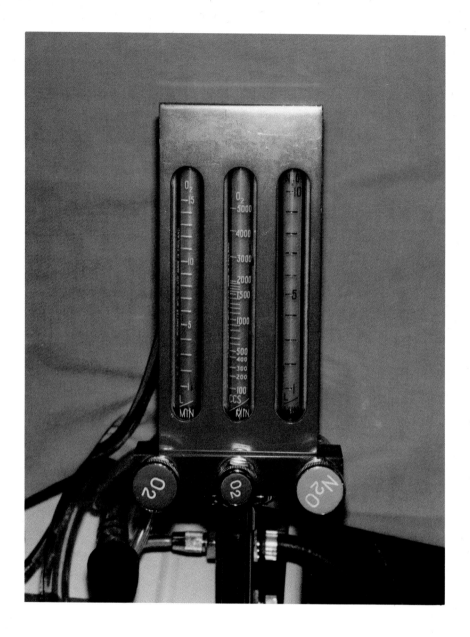

Figure 11 / Flow meter of Engström ventilator. Note non-standard colour of oxygen control knob (blue) and nitrous oxide (green).

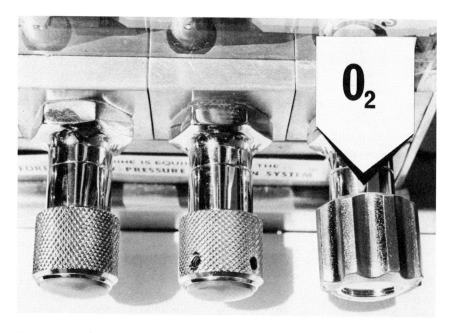

Figure 13 / Flowmeter panel with control knobs. The knob for oxygen differs in size and shape from all others.
*From Rendell-Baker (25); courtesy: Anesthesia and Analgesia —
Current Researches*

or six times the amount of the volatile agent intended to be administered. Obviously the wrong flowmeter and scale had been used during the replacement process.

In another instance (4) it was discovered after a machine had been serviced that, with a rotameter setting of 5 litres per minute of oxygen, an actual volume of only 400 ml was being delivered. Somehow a cyclopropane flowmeter had been placed into the oxygen position, the cyclopropane position carrying no flowmeter at all. In another similar case Slater (29) found that with an expected oxygen percentage of 33 per cent, 52 per cent was actually being delivered, with the result that three patients experienced discomfort and had some recollection of the operation. In this case the flowmeter bobbins for oxygen and nitrous oxide had been transposed accidentally, with the result that oxygen was being delivered at a higher flow and nitrous oxide at a lower flow than anticipated.

Slater suggests that rotameter tubes should be removed only by trained personnel, that after maintenance service the oxygen concentration delivered be checked, and that bobbins be colour-coded. Master flowmeter kits are available to check flowmeters after re-assembly. In Britain bobbins are numbered to correspond with the tube, but in the United States they can be distinguished only by weight. Free movement of the bobbin does not ensure that the actual gas flow is that indicated by its position within the rotameter tube. A prototype pin-index safety system for flowmeter tubes has been developed which would prevent an incorrect tube being used for any particular gas (24). Such flowmeters, indexed to the housing, are fitted to the Chemetron gas machine.

While flowmeters are usually reliable, particles of dust or gummy deposits may enter with the incoming gas, causing the float to stick to the wall. This can give rise to erroneous readings. A particularly dangerous situation can arise if an oxygen flowmeter bobbin sticks (usually at the top of the tube) and at the same time the oxygen supply fails. Clutton-Brock has pointed out that flowmeter inaccuracies are often due to static electricity (5). This may also cause the bobbin to stick and care should therefore be taken to ensure that bobbins keep rotating while in use. If this is not the case a change of gas flow may often distribute the electrical charge from the bobbin over the inside of the glass tube, resulting in its temporary release. Rees has advocated the injection of 1 ml of water into the flowmeter whenever the bobbin stops rotating, a manoeuvre which combats the accumulation of static electricity (23). However Clutton-Brock (6) warns against this practice, pointing out that water settles in the hollow of the bobbin, thus causing even greater inaccuracies. Moreover, water takes a long time to evaporate, thus prolonging the abnormal situation. Manufacturers have now taken steps to reduce the impact of static electricity on flowmeter function by coating the inner surface of the tube with a film of stannous chloride and by application of a ring of gold to the ends of tubes where they make contact with the antistatic rubber bed.

If an obstruction occurs in the low pressure system downstream from the flowmeter and if the system is air-tight, all flowmeter readings will be depressed. If the system is not tight, a leak may develop and the flowmeters remain unchanged despite the reduced flow exhibited to the patient. On the whole, leaks tend to be more common than obstruction, the latter having been eliminated by the substitution of metal for rubber tubing within the anaesthetic machine assembly.

Leakage of gases
Leakage of gases from flowmeters constitutes a major hazard particularly when the leakage is predominantly of oxygen. It is evident from Figure 14 that the danger is aggravated if the oxygen flowmeter is situated upstream in the assembly from the other gases, since more oxygen will be lost, resulting potentially in a hypoxic mixture. This danger is minimized if the oxygen flowmeter is in a downstream position (10). The cause for such leakage may be leaking flowmeter

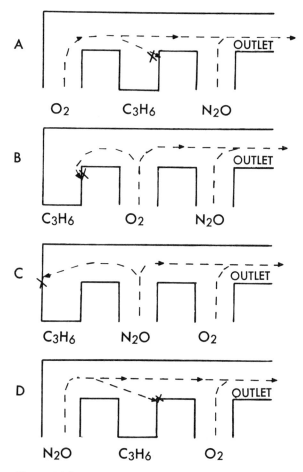

Figure 14 / Four possible three-gas flowmeter sequences. In each case a leak
has developed in the cyclopropane flowmeter tube as indicated by the cross.
Direction of flow of oxygen and nitrous oxide is indicated by the broken arrows.
Configurations A and B are dangerous since oxygen is lost proximal to other
gases; configurations C and D are safe as nitrous oxide, not oxygen, is lost.
From Eger et al. (10); *courtesy: Anesthesiology*

tubes, usually the result of breakage (9). Such a break may be in the form of a
hairline crack which is not immediately visible to the naked eye and can only be
detected by disassembling the entire block (2). However, there may be other
causes for such loss. For instance, Gupta and Varshneya (12) have described loss
of oxygen through a worn sealing washer at the top of the carbon dioxide

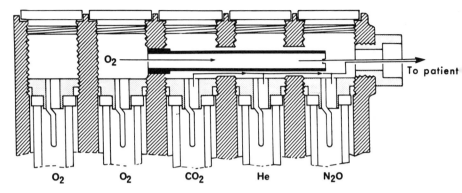

Figure 15 / Modification of Dräger flowmeter assembly with upstream oxygen flowmeter. Insertion of a guide tube into the head of the assembly passes the oxygen direct to the outlet thus bypassing other flowmeters and preventing retrograde loss of oxygen in case of a leak.
From Katz (14); *courtesy: Anesthesia and Analgesia – Current Researches*

rotameter tube. In their case filling of the reservoir bag was inappropriately slow and compression of the bag produced loss of gas. Although a number of episodes of cyanosis ensued, their patient fortunately recovered. This report has been widely commented upon (25, 32). For instance Muliyil (20), in commenting on it, makes the point that service engineers and hospitals in India will be provided with a plug-in manometer with a pre-set pressure-relief valve. Noting the time required for the pressure to increase at a set flow of oxygen, it can be determined whether leaks are present in the system. Similar observations can also be made after the oxygen has been turned off. The manufacturer is to be commended on this initiative which might well be emulated by others. All other correspondents urge that the oxygen flowmeter be moved to the extreme right of the bank or alternatively that baffle systems or a guide tube for oxygen be incorporated to direct the oxygen flow to the outlet of the assembly. Such a relatively simple internal modification, made by Draegerwerk to their flowmeter housing, will neutralize the disadvantages inherent in the upstream position of oxygen flowmeters (14). This consists of a guide tube within the flowmeter assembly which carries the oxygen direct to the outlet of the flowmeter bank past all other flowmeters (Fig. 15). Despite such ingenious modifications, the ultimate solution must be agreement on a standard position for the oxygen flowmeter within the assembly, irrespective of the manufacturer or country of origin. Instinctive identification of oxygen flowmeters by position is as vital as the standard relation of accelerator to brake pedals on motor cars.

Loss of gas from the flowmeter assembly may also occur at a site remote from the flowmeter itself. For instance Liew (16) has drawn attention to the loss of oxygen down a third flowmeter, the gas leaking out in retrograde fashion when the flowmeter needle valve of the third gas is left open and a dummy cylinder block has not been inserted into the yoke. This is prone to happen when the third flowmeter is for cyclopropane or carbon dioxide since, as a rule, no pressure regulator is interposed in the line to block the retrograde flow of gas. A loss of 2 per cent of oxygen by this mechanism was demonstrated when a Magill circuit was used and this increased to 8 per cent with a ventilator. A similar loss of oxygen occurred in a machine modified for the inclusion of air in the gas mixture (17). The air flow control valve was placed remote from the flowmeter, between it and the yoke set aside to receive the supply of air. Oxygen leakage occurred if the compressed air supply was disconnected and the control valve left open (Fig. 16). Katz (13) has described another such incident in which there was a loose connector in the line between the helium flowmeter and a closed remote flow control device, so that oxygen could escape in a retrograde fashion (Fig. 17). With 4-litre flows of oxygen and of nitrous oxide, the mixture issuing from the machine contained only 2 per cent oxygen.

Faults in construction

In some of the older rotameter blocks the bobbin disappears from view when it reaches the upper end of the tube, being obscured by the frame of the flowmeter assembly. In two instances in which the carbon dioxide flowmeter was involved this has led to severe hypercarbia (22, 27). The diagnosis was made in one instance because the absorber got unduly hot twice in quick succession and in the other case hypercarbia was diagnosed by blood gas analysis. A similar instance of a bobbin becoming 'invisible' at a high flow setting has been described by Dinnick (7).

In order to prevent the bobbin of the flowmeter from rising out of sight, the incorporation of a wire coil, a plastic or a rubber buffer have been suggested (31) or else the flowmeter should be constructed in such a way as to give visual access to the flowmeter column in its entire range. This type of construction has been adopted in all newer flowmeter assemblies.

Lomanto and Leeming (18) have described a simple visual warning device in case of excessive gas flows. A lightweight aluminum pin in an air-tight lucite chamber is attached to the top of each flow column. If the bobbin comes in contact with the pin, it is pushed up revealing a bright red top.

Although relating to an oxygen therapy flowmeter rather than to anaesthetic machines as such, it might be mentioned here that Richardson (26) has found

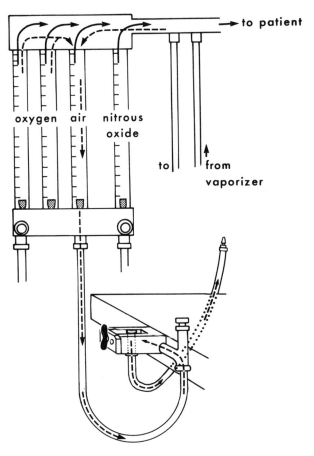

Figure 16 / With the air supply hose disconnected from the source and
the needle valve between yoke and flowmeter open, retrograde leakage occurs
in the direction of the broken arrows.
From Liew and Garmendran (17); courtesy: British Journal of Anaesthesia

that the spur which is intended to prevent the bobbin on the Vickers-Puritan
flowmeter from blocking the exit office on the top of the flowmeter has been
known to break off, thus allowing the exit hole to be closed off by the bobbin.
The higher the flow the more certain is the occlusion. However, this complication is likely to arise only in older type flowmeters since a seat was developed in
1970 by the manufacturers which obviates the need for a spring-type ball stop
(21).

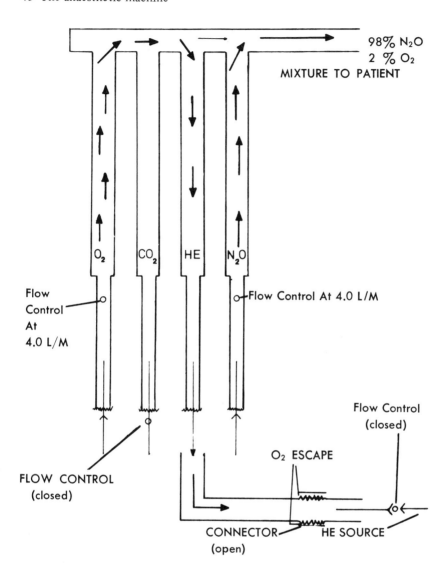

Figure 17 / Loss of oxygen down the helium flowmeter results in delivery of a hypoxic mixture if the helium flow control is closed and the connector is not air-tight.

From Katz (14); courtesy: Anesthesia and Analgesia – Current Researches

Flowmeters may also stick at the bottom with the bobbin hidden, yet with some gas being allowed to flow. If this happens with a flowmeter for an anaesthetic gas, a serious situation can arise.

It may be worthwhile relating an unusual case which occurred with a machine that is no longer being manufactured but of which a few specimens may still be in use. The rotameter bobbin of a Chicago Anesthesia Equipment Company machine behaved erratically when oxygen flow exceeded 5 l/min and a flow of 6 to 8 l/min could not be obtained consistently. When the machine was dismantled a small metal sphere was found at the first coupling connecting the outflow of the oxygen flowmeter to the internal copper tubing system of the machine. This metal sphere acted as a ball valve and at high flow the turbulence of the gas in the coupling would propel the shot into the central gas stream where it impinged upon the opening in the coupling of the tubing. The origin of the shot was traced to a flowmeter bobbin into the hollow of which a shot was cemented; in this case one of these shots had become detached (1).

Miscellaneous accidents

Edwards and associates (9) in a report on deaths associated with anaesthesia include two instances of lethal carbon dioxide concentrations. In one case the same flowmeter had been used for cyclopropane and carbon dioxide, the flow of the latter being controlled by a tap which was accidentally knocked open. In the other case an empty carbon dioxide cylinder was replaced while the flowmeter control valve was still open from a previous case. A flowmeter control valve should always be closed when the flowmeter is not in use.

Some older anaesthetic machines have separate flowmeters for tank and pipeline oxygen, a situation not devoid of danger. A representative case may serve to illustrate this:

A 54-year-old woman was booked for removal of an intracranial haemangioma in the temporo-parietal region. It was customary to induce anaesthesia for neuro-surgical patients in the corridor, so that shaving of the head would not take place in the operating room itself with the inherent danger of contamination. There being no pipeline outlets outside, the operating room cylinder oxygen was used; but after the machine had been moved into the operating room it was then connected to the piped oxygen. However the anaesthetist forgot to open the pipeline oxygen flowmeter and continued with the cylinder flowmeter, not noticing that in due course the cylinder ran empty, resulting in a period of hypoxia. Luckily the error was detected in time and no harm came to the patient.

Another example of duplicated flowmeters is that of the side-by-side existence of fine and coarse calibration oxygen flowmeters. Here again a potential danger is the erroneous use of the wrong flowmeter and the following case illustrates that particular situation:

A 54-year-old woman was scheduled for cystoscopy and change of ureteral catheter. Five minutes after induction of anaesthesia cyanosis was first noted and in due course became more marked. The resident being unable to determine the cause called his consultant who flushed the system with oxygen thus restoring a good colour. On subsequent examination of the machine it was found that while the nitrous oxide was flowing at 8 l/min the fine flow oxygen flowmeter was used at 200 ml/min rather than the intended 2 l/min on the coarse flow one. Again the situation was remedied before serious harm befell the patient.

Mazze (19) had a similar experience. The unfortunate outcome in his case underlines the potential danger of such dual flowmeter arrangements.

Copper kettles are highly accurate vaporizers, but since each requires its own flowmeter, the array of flowmeters becomes impressive if more than one kettle is installed. It requires experience and concentration to operate such a machine safely and effectively. Complex flowmeter arrangements obviously invite errors and so does the manner in which flows are marked on the flowmeter tube. Where the same flowmeter combines high and low oxygen flow graduations it is always possible for millilitres to be misread for litre flows, with consequent administration of hypoxic mixtures. Spoerel (30) has witnessed such an occurrence and so has the author.

Because of all these instances of actual or potential hypoxia, the suggestion by Mazze (19) that in-line oxygen monitors be installed has much merit.

While their use in connection with anaesthesia is infrequent, nevertheless a warning is necessary against small flowmeters since they have been known to explode if no reducing valve is fitted (8).

VAPORIZERS

Vaporizer inaccuracies
Since the introduction of halothane, precision temperature-compensated vaporizers have come into general use for all new inhalation agents. The most commonly-used vaporizers for halothane are the Fluotec, the copper kettle, of which the Vernitrol is an adaptation, and the Dräger-Vapor.

In contrast to less complicated appliances, many of the new sophisticated vaporizers are in need of periodic maintenance. In the case of the Fluotec, for instance, this involves cleaning the spindle and wick which becomes partly clogged with the thymol in the halothane, and periodic recalibration by the manufacturer. After use, many vaporizers have been found to deliver small amounts of halothane even at the zero setting, an important consideration if one subscribes to the theory of sensitization to halothane which, in that case, may well take place inadvertently in the course of an anaesthetic in which apparently no halothane has been administered (30). Morgan and Lumley (25) have found that in vaporizers not serviced for an unknown duration there was a tendency at a fresh flow of 8 l/min to get high concentrations at low dial settings with the Fluotec Mark II and lower concentrations at high dial settings, with the change-over taking place approximately at the two per cent level; this contradicts an earlier paper (24) in which they had stated that after use for one year there was no deterioration in performance in most of the vaporizers tested which, in addition to the Fluotec Mark II, included the *M.I.E. Halothane IV*. Murray and Fleming (28) have found that between the OFF and the 0.2 per cent dial setting of the Fluotec Mark II there is little difference in concentration delivered at a 6 l/min gas flow. Hill (14) has confirmed that errors in dial calibration are greater at low flow rates and at low vapour percentages.

Hall and associates (13) have compared the simple, small but inefficient *Goldman vaporizer* with the large, complicated but highly efficient Fluotec. They again confirm that, in the case of the Fluotec, concentrations in excess of low dial settings are being delivered, whereas with high settings concentrations are below expectations. Indeed, in one instance only 2.4 per cent was obtained at the 4 per cent setting. Prolonged use, that is two runs of one hour each, did not affect results. These authors feel that in actual clinical practice it is not necessary to be able to vary concentrations by accurately known small amounts and hence would prefer the Goldman vaporizer which, because of its simplicity, is less prone to failure or accidental overdose, if it could be constructed in such a way as to be capable of delivering concentrations of up to 5 per cent. Adner and Hallen (1) who tested 10 Mark II Fluotecs of different ages and at different dial settings and oxygen flows by means of gas chromatography found considerable divergences and even some overlapping between these different dial settings. None gave the concentrations they were supposed to give and deviations were often more than 50 per cent of expected value. They found these inaccuracies to be related to the age of the vaporizer and indeed a new one tested by them gave quite acceptable values.

However, there are yet other sources of inaccuracy. For instance, with a Fluotec Mark II outside the circle during assisted or controlled ventilation in either closed or semi-closed circuits, halothane concentrations delivered are significantly increased above the percentage indicated on the calibration curves, as a result of pressure fluctuations within the circuit (15, 17). Errors due to this pumping effect can be prevented by the interposition of a check valve which, of course, must be completely competent and which must be large enough and close enough to the anaesthetic circuit to minimize resistance to gas flow. Such valves are now fitted on new vaporizers. In the Dräger 'vapor' a tube capacitor is used for this purpose rather than a check-valve (34). This arrangement is equally effective and indeed more foolproof. Fluctuations can be further reduced by the use of a 0.5 litre collecting bag for use with low flow techniques. Kapfhammer and Atabas (16) have proven that a pressure equilibrating valve placed into the outlet of the Fluotec will also prevent inaccuracies arising with low fresh gas flows during assisted or controlled ventilation. Gordh and associates (9) have confirmed that deviations from preset concentrations occur during intermittent positive pressure ventilation also with the Engström ventilator and again these inaccuracies are more significant at small volumes. Indeed cyclic pressure changes within the ventilator are reflected in the pressures within the vaporizer. There is every possibility that flow through the vaporizer may vary in amount and direction with pressure changes in the ventilator so that certain proportions of gas may pass through the vaporizer more than once.

The increase in halothane output during intermittent positive pressure is not limited to the Fluotec in the absence of a check valve, but also applies to the *Vernitrol* as shown by Eger (6). However, he believes that this is of relatively little importance compared to the increased input of halothane into the alveoli occasioned by the increased ventilation. Keet, Valentine, and Riccio (18) recommend the addition of a check valve inside the machine in preference to one placed externally, since this would isolate the vaporizer from the diluent as well as the circle gas. Eger agrees that such an internal check valve provides absolute protection against the increased halothane output from a Vernitrol during intermittent positive pressure but, of course, neither the external nor the internal check valve will protect against the increased input of halothane into the alveoli. Even with no check valve the maximum rise in concentration is only 0.6 per cent higher than expected, corresponding to a 0.25 per cent rise in inspired concentration in a closed circuit (19). Mulroy, Ham, and Eger (26) have recently seen machine failures which might have caused the delivery of hypoxic mixtures. In each case the O-ring in the on-off mechanism of the side-arm Vernitrol was broken. Since hitherto no protection has been incorporated against back pressure in the outlet line, such breakage is likely to be a source of a leak of anaesthetic gases when positive pressure ventilation is used. A check valve has been developed and this should be installed in all older models; it is now standard on all new side-arm Vernitrols. This will prevent a leak of 'diluent gases' into the circuit from the common manifold, but unless placed in the proper position may still allow escape of oxygen-vapour mixture from the leaking valve. This results in selective loss of the vaporized agent rather than in hypoxia (7).

A Heidbrink series DM 5000 Kinet-O-Meter with *heated vaporizer kettles* and flowmeters calibrated in volumes of vapour rather than oxygen was found to deliver halothane when the flush valve was operated with the halothane vaporizer shunt valve open and with no oxygen being directed through the vaporizer. This did not occur with the shunt valve closed (11). This vaporizer is protected against back pressure within the kettle during intermittent positive pressure ventilation at low flows by means of a spring-loaded valve intended to keep a pressure of approximately 40 torr (5.3 kPa) within the vaporizer. In this particular machine the pressure was 58-60 torr (7.7-8 kPa) and rose to 94-112 torr (12.5-14.9 kPa) on flushing with the shunt valve on. As flushing ceased and the pressure fell rapidly to 60 torr (8 kPa) again, oxygen containing up to 3.1 per cent halothane vapour was released into the delivery hose.

Rendell-Baker (32) has drawn attention to a serious flaw inherent in the concept of the combined oxygen flush-vaporizer on/off tap used with the kettle type vaporizer. If induction of anaesthesia is with an agent of low vapour pressure, such as methoxyflurane, it may be necessary to use the patient's total oxygen requirement as the carrier gas. If, after using the oxygen flush, the anaesthetist fails to turn on the vaporizer again, the carrier gas in its entirety will be vented to atmosphere and no oxygen reaches the patient. Hence some machines have been designed so that the oxygen flush valve and vaporizer shunt valve are controlled by the same lever, requiring the shunt valve to be off before flushing can begin. This is a safety measure which should be encouraged, but such a lever is not part of the machine under discussion.

The now obsolete *Gardner Universal Vaporizer* has been tested by Weis and Schreiber (37). This was a vaporizer with an ingeniously constructed exchangeable key allowing it to be used with a number of volatile anaesthetics. It could serve as a draw-over vaporizer or as part of an anaesthetic machine. Unfortunately the concentration measured bore little resemblance to the key setting and this was corroborated by Tammisto (36) who found the function of twelve out of sixteen vaporizers unsatisfactory. Only four were found acceptable, with an accuracy of ±20 per cent at steady gas flows over a range of three to ten l/min. These findings applied both to use in standard push-over configuration and to the draw-over technique, while all were found to function inadequately when intermittent positive pressure ventilation was used. Although this particular vaporizer was not found acceptable because of its unreliable performance characteristics, it must also be said that a universal vaporizer is undesirable in principle since there is always the danger that residues of a previously used anaesthetic may remain to contaminate a subsequently used agent or that a wrong key may be used for the agent being administered and thus lead to concentrations that bear no relation to the dial setting. Any universal vaporizers must be rejected for that reason alone.

The *Oxford miniature vaporizer* (OMV) for halothane has been designed for use with the Oxford inflating bellows in a draw-over system. Under these conditions the concentration delivered depends on the velocity of the gas flow produced by the expansion of the breathing bag which takes about one second. The delivered halothane concentration corresponds well with the dial setting on the vaporizer. In contrast, if the Ambu-Ruben bag, which expands in approximately 0.3 seconds, is used with this vaporizer, the halothane output is significantly reduced because of the higher gas flow and its shorter exposure to the liquid anaesthetic. If used in a push-over configuration, the performance of this vaporizer is influenced by lung compliance and by the properties of certain components of the anaesthesia circuit such as valves and rubber components and the delivered halothane concentration is always greater than that indicated on the dial setting. In some instances the increase has amounted to 0.5 to 1.0 vol per cent (12).

Errors in the use of vaporizers
One of the most common errors associated with the use of vaporizers is the *contamination of downstream in-series vaporizers* (29, 38). This is most likely to occur when a vaporizer designed for a low vapour pressure anaesthetic is placed downstream from one intended for use with a higher vapour pressure — likely because both vaporizers are opened simultaneously, either accidentally or on purpose (Fig. 18). Contamination of methoxyflurane by halothane under these conditions has been found in 70 per cent of vaporizers tested and in two of them the concentrations were quite high. Consequently, halothane may be delivered unintentionally together with the methoxyflurane in concentrations which in themselves may be in the anaesthetic range, depending upon the degree of contamination and the setting of the vaporizer. It is evident that this can lead to serious clinical complications. Contamination of vaporizers can be prevented by placing them in parallel rather than in series. The 'Selectatec' vaporizer attachment bar (Fraser Sweatman Inc.) is useful in this regard since it prevents two vaporizers from being used simultaneously. A similar system is available also on the Dräger machine (32) in the form of 'Selector' switches. In the new Chemetron gas machine, this same problem has been solved by the provision of a flexible hose between flowmeter block outlet and vaporizer inlet. Thus only one vaporizer can be connected at any given time.

Another problem is the inadvertent filling of a vaporizer with the wrong anaesthetic. In the course of a seminar on 'Safety in the Operating Room', anaesthetists were asked to detect by smell the presence of halothane with which a 'Pentec' vaporizer had been filled (31). They could not do this successfully since the more pungent smell of the residual methoxyflurane masked that of halothane. This observation confirms once again that should a Pentec inadvertently be filled with the more volatile halothane, a very dangerous situation could exist, since up to 30 per cent halothane could be delivered by a Pentec vaporizer so filled in error. A fatal case in which a kettle vaporizer had been filled erroneously

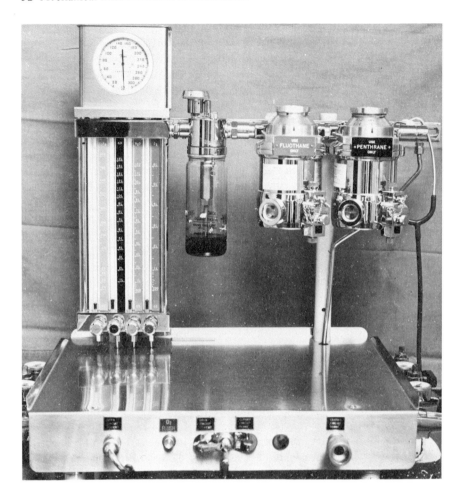

Figure 18 / Pentec vaporizer in downstream position in relation to Fluotec on a Canadian Heidbrink machine. This machine had been in daily use for a number of years.

with trichlorethylene instead of halothane has been described by Chun and Karp (3). The adoption of a pin-index system for vaporizers is strongly recommended and has been in use in Canada for a number of years (2). Yet this system too can fail as its cousin for cylinders has also done on occasion. McBurney has reported such an instance in which the receptacle for halothane was found to accept the filling device for enflurane, probably because the pin inside the receptacle was too small or had been worn down permitting insertion, although the groove on the filler head was not in line with the pin (23).

Delivery of liquid anaesthetic is a complication of the greatest gravity, often leading to cardio-vascular collapse.

Many of the copper kettle vaporizers in use have the filling port on the top, which may lead to overfilling and consequent delivery of liquid anaesthetic. This can be prevented by transposing the filler to the side of the vaporizer at the maximum safe filling level. Liquid halothane has been known to enter the breathing tube on the outlet side if a free-standing Fluotec vaporizer was tipped even fleetingly (27).

Kopriva and Lowenstein (20) found that in two of five of their machines the Vernitrol vaporizer was capable of delivering liquid halothane when the flowmeter bobbin was at the top of the flowmeter and the vaporizer was filled to the 'maximum safe level' mark. The source of this malfunction was traced to a damaged flowmeter needle valve seat which caused the bobbin to move through the entire halothane flowmeter range with only a one-quarter turn of the control knob. Further turning of the control knob then led to the delivery of liquid halothane. The manufacturer later supplied a limiting orifice in the oxygen delivery line to the vaporizer which limited the flow to 900 ml/min to avoid such an occurrence.

Liquid halothane has also been known to cascade from the 'Side-arm Vernitrol' into its flowmeter when the breathing bag was compressed, because of a loose hex-nut cap on the flowmeter tubes. This provides an avenue for escape of pressure on the rotameter side of the circuit. Under normal circumstances the compensating pressure within the flowmeter prevents such backflow (8).

The 'Flow-Critical' Foregger trichlorethylene vaporizer will empty its content in liquid form within two seconds if gas is allowed to flow through it in the reverse direction to that intended. This may occur because this particular vaporizer is designed to be attached to a male 15-mm common gas outlet of the Foregger machine while most other modern machines are provided with female common gas outlets (32).

One further source of liquid anaesthetic has been identified by DeGuzman and Cascorbi (5). Application of as little as 17 ppm of Dow-Corning No. 11 sealant to the copper kettle will deliver foamy or liquid methoxyflurane in the presence of oxygen. Similar observations had been made previously by others and have been confirmed by Sweatman (35) who emphasized that this hazard can be avoided entirely by the use of wick rather than bubble-through vaporizers. In the laboratory, foaming will occur with only 0.004 mg in 100 gm of methoxyflurane. The same phenomenon has been shown to occur with trichlorethylene and chloroform but not with other inhalation agents (21).

Overfilling, short of causing delivery of liquid anaesthetic, has been known to affect the concentration of the agent. A vaporizer, since withdrawn from the market, was found to deliver three to four times the indicated concentration when filled only 4 mm above the 'full' line, since this caused bubbling of the carrier gas through the halothane (33).

Miscellaneous observations

While the control on top of the Fluotec vaporizer reduces the concentration of the agent or turns it off by clockwise rotation, the Foregger and Dräger vaporizers do so by anti-clockwise rotation (Fig. 19 A-D). This constitutes an unnecessary hazard (32).

That malfunctions of vaporizers are not limited to the sophisticated ones is illustrated by the following case:

A one-year-old child was being anaesthetized for ventriculogram, followed by the insertion of a ventriculo-peritoneal shunt. It had been the intention to use a nitrous oxide-relaxant sequence for maintenance of anaesthesia, but it became evident that the level of anaesthesia was too light. Consequently azeotrope halothane-ether was added to the anaesthetic from the ether bottle of a Boyle anaesthetic machine. Immediately thereafter the machine was found to deliver an inadequate flow of gas to the patient and although all common sources of leaks were checked, none were found. As soon as the vaporizer had been turned off again, an adequate gas flow was restored to the patient. Closer inspection of the glass vaporizer bottle confirmed the presence of a washer but this was found to be somewhat more prominent on one side and consequently the bottle was unscrewed. This revealed that the washer had been placed eccentrically, a fact which accounted for the substantial leak as soon as the vaporizer was included into the breathing circuit (Fig. 20 A, B). Since it had not been the anaesthetist's intention to use an inhalation supplement, the circuit had not been checked for air-tightness with the vaporizer included in it.

Special care must be taken that vaporizers not permanently attached to a machine are connected properly to the circuit when placed into use. We have one case on record in our department in which the Pentec vaporizer was incorporated into the Magill circuit of the machine while the circle system was actually being used. In another case a vaporizer was short-circuited entirely out of the delivery system. Neither of these errors was potentially dangerous but, of course, it was impossible to maintain adequate depth of anaesthesia. On the other hand, a hazardous situation arises if the Cyprane vaporizer is set up in reverse manner, as the concentration delivered is approximately double that indicated on the dial. This vaporizer allows flow in the reverse direction, and wrong connection is facilitated by the fact that labelling of inlet and outlet ports is not conspicuous and tubes fit both (22).

Gorgerino, Gazzano, and Vassoney (10) have pointed out that at high altitudes the boiling point of halothane is considerably lower than at sea level and different vaporizers deliver higher concentrations than indicated for dial settings up to two per cent.

Finally even an 'explosion' in a vaporizer has been described by Cohen and Groveman (4). This rather strange accident occurred when the pin controlling the motion of a shunt valve at the 'on' and 'flush' position in the anaesthetic machine was sheared off by vigorous turning. This allowed the valve to go from the 'off' position past the 'flush' far enough for the vent to the copper kettle vaporizer to open. When oxygen was flushed, the build-up of pressure resulted in a blow-out at the weakest point of the system, the glass window of the vaporizer.

FAIL-SAFE SYSTEMS

Since this book deals with equipment failures, it is proper to say a few words about fail-safe and similar devices which have been conceived to safeguard the patient from unrecognized failure of the oxygen supply in the course of an anaesthetic. Only brief mention will be made of this subject since we are primarily concerned with situations of supply and equipment failure rather than with the precise mechanisms designed to forestall such failures or remedy their consequences.

Mere observation of pressure gauges, flowmeters, the breathing bag, and the patient himself should alert the anaesthetist to failure of gas supply. Oxygen supply failure may be indicated by an alarm, visual or auditory or both, or by a true fail-safe device which in the event of failing oxygen pressure is supposed automatically to shut off the supply of nitrous oxide or other anaesthetic or inert gases, venting the system to atmosphere (18). For details of the mechanics of the numerous solutions which have been suggested in the past and of those which are commercially available the reader is referred to the literature (1-7, 9-17, 20-26).

None of these safety devices is totally reliable and the devices themselves have been known to fail. This is a particularly dangerous situation since their very installation on the machines suggests that deprivation of oxygen because of supply failures will not occur. Consequently, in the rare event that this should happen and the warning system should fail, no suspicion will be aroused as to

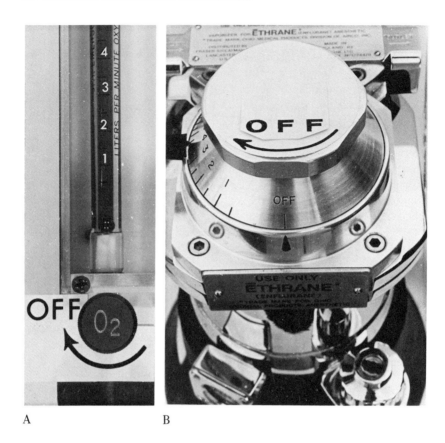

A   B

Figure 19 / A and B, the flowmeter and Ethrane vaporizer, close by clockwise
rotation, whereas C and D, the Foregger Penthrane and the Dräger Vapor
Halothane vaporizers, close by anti-clockwise rotation.
From Rendell-Baker (24); *courtesy: Anesthesia and Analgesia –*
Current Researches

the reason for the deterioration of the patient's condition (27). Furthermore
some devices are inoperative in the presence of artificial ventilation of an
apnoeic patient (8, 19), and others can be inactivated intentionally. For instance
the 'Bosun' oxygen failure alarm has a tap to disconnect it and its whistle, and a
switch to extinguish the alarm light.

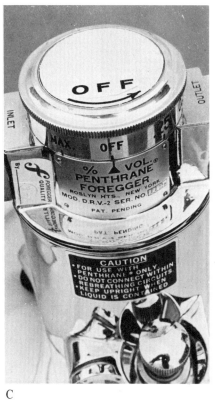

C

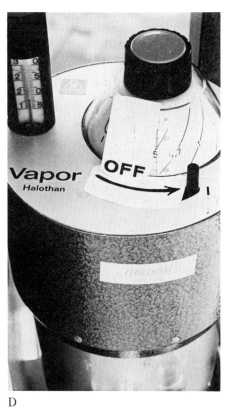

D

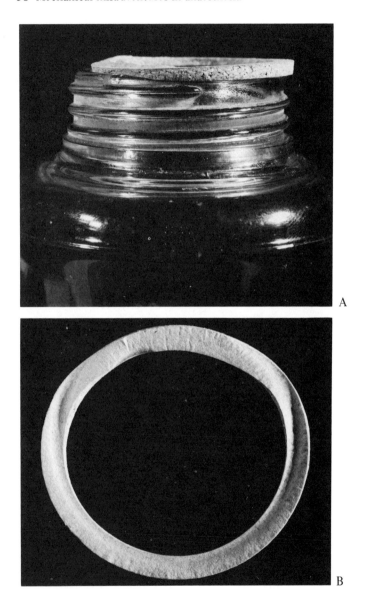

Figure 20 / A, Eccentric position of gasket atop the vaporizer bottle; B, indentation on gasket.

IV
The breathing system

GENERAL CONSIDERATIONS

Many kinds of malfunction or causes of complications are so obvious that they should not need special emphasis. Clearly, care must be taken that all controls on the machine are set properly at all times and that adjustments are made whenever necessary. Only through continuous observation of the flowmeters for instance is it possible to recognize when gas supplies become exhausted. Personnel in the operating room must be dissuaded from leaning against any part of the anaesthetic machine lest they inadvertently interfere with the controls. In one case in our department gas flow had become diverted accidentally from the Magill to the circle system in the course of an anaesthetic, probably by the unwitting interference of a third person. The two-way tap for trichlorethylene on the Boyle machine can be similarly interferred with. It also goes without saying that vaporizer filler ports must be securely closed after filling; failure to observe this precaution has led to many difficulties in maintaining adequate anaesthesia. A particular problem has been encountered with the filler cap on the back of the Ohio DM-5000 vaporizer (8). This cap had a tendency to loosen spontaneously, allowing gas to escape. The problem has now been solved by changing the type of plastic used in the manufacture of the cap. Furthermore, copper kettle and Vernitrol shunt valves must be opened if these vaporizers are expected to deliver anaesthetic vapours into the system.

A good working knowledge of the machine and its parts and their purpose is essential if major errors in use are to be avoided, as illustrated below:

A young boy undergoing repair of an inguinal hernia in a small country hospital died because the physician administering the anaesthetic excluded the 're-breathing bag' from the Magill circuit since he had heard in a lecture that re-breathing was bad in paediatric anaesthesia.

In contrast the breathing bag was kept in the system in another case brought to our attention, while a Manley ventilator was being used. This combination results in the bag getting bigger and bigger whereas the lungs are not being ventilated.

Mention should be made that in assembling the breathing system provision must be made to prevent gases from entering the airway under unmodified high pressure. Edwards and associates (9) found that no less than three times in 1,000 deaths oxygen had been administered under pressure directly to the tracheal tube without the benefit of any intervening moderating device such as a pressure relief valve, resulting each time in mediastinal emphysema. Likewise, care must be taken when inflating the lungs with an Ayre-T-piece by means of intermittent occlusion of the open end that flow rates are such that unduly high pressures are not produced in the system. A case is on record (1) in which a pneumothorax was caused because the flush valve was activated in a three-months old child while the open end of the T-piece was being occluded to inflate the lungs. The danger of this practice becomes obvious if one considers that in doing so one delivers a flow of 60 to 65 litres per minute directly to the tracheal tube with no exit provided. Several other causes of overpressure have been recorded (6), including non-compliant reservoir bags, sticking, faulty, or absent expiratory valves, incorrect assembly of circuit components, etc. Many of these causes will be discussed in detail elsewhere in the appropriate context.

Brière, Patoine, and Audet (2) have drawn attention to an arrangement which they found in a number of Boyle anaesthetic machines (Model M 222) in which the fresh gas inlet into the circle was on the patient side of the inspiratory valve (Fig. 21). While this arrangement in itself is not harmful, it does interfere with the use of a ventilation meter on the expiratory limb of the circuit since the meter will not only record the exhaled volume of gas but also any fresh gas input which continues to flow during exhalation and which incidentally passes out of the surplus gas relief valve without ever reaching the patient.

Mention has been made elsewhere (p. 6) of the necessity of testing all equipment before use. In the case of a closed system, it is imperative that the exclusion of leaks in the low pressure system be assured. Whitcher et al. (12) advise sealing the system, adding gas to the circuit until 30 cm H_2O (5.4 kPa) pressure is reached within the circuit and then observing the pressure. Gas is added as needed and this indicates the size of the leak from the circuit. Dorsch and Dorsch (7) recommend setting a flow of 1 l/min on the oxygen flowmeter and occluding the machine outlet or delivery hose. If the float in the flowmeter drops, any leak in the system is less than 1 l/min. Smaller leaks are detected better by Witcher's method. Page (10) connects a pressure gauge to the common gas outlet or to the patient end of the breathing system. The oxygen is then turned on slowly and the flow stabilized at a level at which the manometer reads a steady 120 mmHg (15 kPa). The volume measured on the rotameter represents the leak. Debban and Bedford (5) have observed that when the occluding thumb was removed from the mask outlet white material, shown to be soda-lime dust, was observed issuing from the face mask. This presumably had been shaken loose and deposited in the inspiratory limb of the circuit whence it had been blown out. Dust and particles can accumulate in the base of the soda-lime absorber as a result of vibrations when the machine is moved from place to place. There are four ways in which this hazard can be avoided. Either the bag should be placed on the inspiratory side of the circuit, or it should be only partially filled and lightly squeezed and released without build-up of great pressure in the system followed by sudden release, or else venting should be through the pop-off valve on the expiratory side of the anaesthesia circuit rather than the mask opening. Lastly, wetting of the soda lime will also solve the problem. Ribak (11) has been unable to reproduce the findings just quoted with pre-packed disposable tandem carbon dioxide absorber canisters. This would appear to be another solution of the problem.

A relatively new set of complications has been introduced by the widespread use of disposable breathing components. These complications have included kinking and indentation into the lumen of breathing tubes, breakage of connectors, separation of the swivel connector, and leaks at connector sites or along breathing tubes (3). Trace anaesthetic gas concentrations in the anaesthetist's breathing zone have been found to be well above target levels when swivel-type disposable circuits were used, despite gas scavenging devices and adequate fresh air exchange rates in the operating room. Concentrations were lower when Y-type disposable connectors were used (4).

While both the anaesthetic machine and the breathing system may be functioning perfectly well, errors may be made in joining them together. The following case is a good example of such an error:

A 66-year-old woman was anaesthetized in routine fashion and anaesthesia was maintained with a circle absorber in a Boyle machine of the kind which has separate common gas outlets for the Magill and the circle systems. Shortly after maintenance had become established, the expiratory hose of the circle system became detached from the machine. It was immediately re-inserted but accidently not into the port from which it had come but rather into the common gas outlet for the Magill circuit. This, of course, resulted in

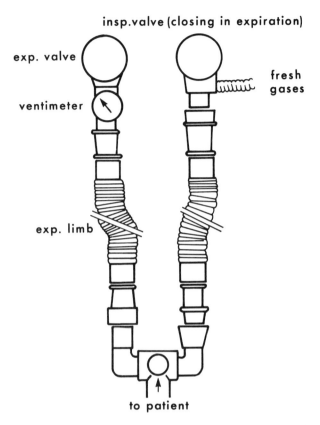

Figure 21 / With the fresh gas inlet on the inspiratory side of the circuit
the ventimeter records both the expiratory volume and the fresh gases flowing
during exhalation.
From Brière, Patoine and Audet (2); *courtesy: Canadian Anaesthetists'
Society Journal*

complete blockage of gas return and over-distention of the lungs. Before the error
was detected and rectified, cardiac arrest had ensued from which, however, the
patient was easily resuscitated and fortunately there were no long-term ill effects.

In another case of improper connection, the Marrett anaesthetic machine was
involved. This machine called for an occluding plug to be inserted into the
expiratory limb of the circle system if a Magill or similar circuit was to be used
which was then attached to the inspiratory limb:

A six-day-old infant was to undergo an operation for congenital glaucoma. Tracheal intubation was carried out awake and an Ayre-T-piece was attached to the tracheal tube. Despite increasing concentrations of anaesthetic agents, the infant would not go to sleep and in order to hasten the induction, the free limb of the T-piece was occluded intermittently with each inspiratory effort. In due course respiration became shallow and jerky, accompanied by increasing pallor. All anaesthetics were discontinued and mouth-to-mouth respiration was instituted. By this time heart sounds had disappeared and open thoracotomy was done. The heart was re-started immediately, and since spontaneous respiration had resumed, the patient was allowed to breathe spontaneously. The baby never seemed to be anaesthetized properly throughout the short procedure which otherwise proceeded uneventfully. It was only later when an adult was to be anaesthetized with the same machine that it was realized that the circuit had been connected to the expiratory port of the Marrett head with the inspiratory limb occluded by the plug.

Many other examples of misconnections come to mind, as for instance the interchange of reservoir bag and inspiratory hose, a mistake which is particularly easily made if the bag is mounted on an extension hose. The bag has also been known to be connected to the expiratory side of the system. Another example is the transposition of the bag hose to the hose on the absorber of the MIE machine. Many of these errors can be avoided by assigning specific dimensions to the bag mount, thus making it non-interchangeable with other ports.

BREATHING BAGS, TUBES, AND BACTERIAL FILTERS

Relatively few misadventures can be ascribed to breathing bags, other than leakage because of punctures, tears, or open tails, partial or complete. One case is on record in our department in which difficulty was experienced with ventilating the lungs of a young child. The cause was found to be multiple leaks in the breathing tubes, which had been patched with adhesive tape, aggravated by a hole in the reservoir bag. While it may be necessary to close leaks by adhesive **tape** or generally to improvise for on-the-spot solution of an existing situation, such defective parts must be replaced as soon as possible. Another hazard of old bags is that they may become completely detached from their mount when used for controlled ventilation.

Bags made of thin rubber with the neck held between two rubber collars without vulcanization or adhesive are also hazardous because the bag may become detached during controlled ventilation and cannot be easily replaced.

Lynch (7) found that removal of the stopcock from the tail of certain bags failed to allow escape of excess gas. It was then ascertained that the stopcock is held in position by adhesive, an excess of which caused the walls of the tail to stick together after withdrawal of the stopcock.

Parmley and associates (9) have drawn attention to some early disposable bags made of plastic which were non-distensible. The bags performed well until they were full; then any further gas would generate dangerous pressure. Proposed International Standards Organization standards for bag compliance have been drafted, and bags now available are excellent.

Cozanitis and Takkunen (3) have encountered a rather unique abnormality affecting the tubing of a ventilator. In this case a fold had formed at the junction of the supported and unsupported portions of the tubing of an Engström ventilator leading to aneurysm formation, which in turn obstructed the lumen. In another rare incident (1) a breathing tube for infant use was inserted between the Y-piece and a tracheostomy adaptor of a patient on a ventilator to add deadspace. With the insertion of the breathing tube ventilation became impossible and on investigation it was found that the bushing of the tube was occluded completely by a rubber diaphragm. However, the commonest cause of obstruction is water in breathing tubes.

The largest number of incidents with breathing tubes has occurred since the introduction of the Bain circuit. Most relate to the avulsion of the inner tube from the machine end of the circuit. When this happens, hypercarbia is the inevitable result because of the removal of the fresh gas from the immediate vicinity of the tracheal tube with consequent increase in the deadspace (5, 14). Where the outer tube is transparent this can be checked by inspection, especially if the machine end of the inner tube has been appropriately identified (2). In non-transparent tubes the intactness or otherwise of the inner tube connection may be tested by flushing the system from the oxygen bypass. If the circuit is intact and there is no obstruction, the high velocity flow of gas in the inner tube causes a venturi effect, lowering the pressure in the outer tube, and the reservoir bag consequently collapses. If the inner tube has become disconnected from its mount, however, the reservoir bag will not only fail to collapse, but may indeed inflate slightly (11). A venturi effect can also be created by placing the little finger against the inner wall of the outer tube at its distal end, and at the same time partially occluding the inner tube. Again, a negative pressure is created within the circuit, if it is intact, and the walls of the reservoir bag are drawn together (12). In describing this test, Salt emphasizes that it must be used only if the machine is protected by a relief valve operating at about 51 kPa (60 cm H_2O), since otherwise prolonged occlusion may blow off the inner tube of the Bain circuit or damage the anaesthetic machine. Another test has been described by Foëx and Crampton Smith (4): integrity of the circuit is indicated by a slight descent of the rotameters when the inner tube is occluded by insertion of the index finger into the patient end of the circuit.

Recently the Bureau of Medical Devices of the Health Protection Branch, Department of Health and Welfare for Canada, has circulated an 'Alert' in which it is pointed out that the swivel mount of the Bain breathing circuit attachment, as supplied by one of the manufacturers in Canada, has a 20 mm male/15 mm female coaxial fitting which is identical with that of the common gas outlet. Consequently a misconnection can occur with the result that no fresh gas reaches the inner tube of the Bain attachment and the entire system is thus converted to deadspace with all fresh gas escaping through the exhalation valve located near the machine end of the outer tube. It is precisely to forestall this kind of potential hazard that in future standards the 20 mm male/15 mm female coaxial fitting is going to be reserved exclusively for components carrying gases to the patient, thus making it non-interchangeable with all other connections. In another instance the fresh gas flow line was connected by mistake to the nipple for the pressure manometer of the ventilator while the manometer in turn was connected to the inflow orifice of the Bain tube. Here again the entire outer tube became deadspace with consequent development of hypercarbia, while the fresh gas supply escaped through the valve (10).

Other than disconnection, the inner tube of the Bain circuit can also become kinked (Fig. 22) as described by Mansell (8). It is surmised that the inner tube was cut too long during manufacture, resulting in its kinking when it was accommodated within the outside tube. It is interesting to note that this defect which, of course, occluded completely the inflow of fresh air, was only seen when the circuit was examined over a strong light, despite the transparency of the outer tube. Given these many hazards one wonders whether it might not be wise to attach the fresh gas tube externally to the corrugated tubing.

Be this as it may, co-axial circuits must not be used with demand-type gas machines as resistance of the inner tube may restrict total flow below that needed to prevent rebreathing and because back-pressure may affect the accuracy of the mixture controls (13).

Finally, mention should be made of the role of *bacterial filters* which are frequently interposed in breathing circuits. They should be made of material unaffected by high humidity which otherwise offers increased resistance to breathing. Most filters are intended for single use only and, if re-sterilized, may greatly increase resistance to breathing, a complication which has led to fatalities.

Complete obstruction of an in-line bacterial filter in the expiratory limb of a circle circuit occurred due to pulmonary oedema fluid (6). Fluid is forced into the filter from the patient side, but the filter can be cleared by positive pressure from the opposite side. The inspiratory filter remains functional since any fluid which might have reached it is expelled by the gas flow in the opposite direction. It follows that filters should only be used on the inspiratory limb of a breathing

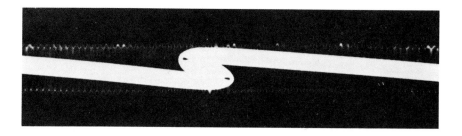

Figure 22 / X-ray of a Bain tube with kinked, obstructed inner tube.
From Mansell (8); *courtesy: Canadian Anaesthetists' Society Journal*

circuit and that an expiratory filter should only be added in cases of active infectious pulmonary disease. Neither should filters on the expiratory side be used in patients subject to pulmonary haemorrhage or oedema.

CARBON DIOXIDE ABSORBERS

Carbon dioxide absorbers are relatively simple devices which consequently do not present too many problems provided they are filled properly and leaks caused by faulty re-assembly after filling are avoided. Most absorbers in common use today are of the circle variety and it is to these that reference will be made in this chapter.

In 1958 and again in 1959 a defect was described in which exhaled gases did not pass through the absorber of some McKesson Model N machines because of a defective by-pass valve. Consequently there was a build-up of carbon dioxide on the inhalation side. The defect was corrected by the manufacturer in due course and since machines of this particular vintage are not likely to be still in use, this particular malfunction is largely of historical interest (6, 7). Another cause of failure of carbon dioxide absorption in an antiquated machine, namely a Chicago Anesthetic Machine canister, was traced to an imperfect seal between the straight middle edge of the baffle plate of the absorber and the edges of the canister. Sealing of the plate edges with caulking compound controlled the malfunction (8).

Danielson (2) has described a potential danger inherent in double canister circle filter heads in which a coupled shunt valve is placed at the bottom of the canister intended to direct the gas flow to one canister or the other. If by mischance this valve is placed at the halfway position, between 'on' and 'off,' then all gases coming from the machine by-pass the breathing bag and are shunted directly to the patient. In this case no relief valve remains in the system

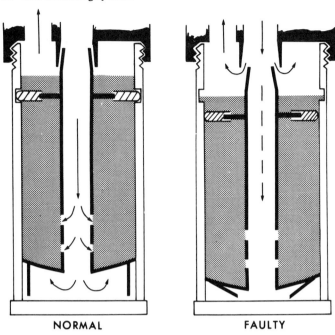

NORMAL   FAULTY

Figure 23 / Normal and faulty condition of MIE Lincoln 800 soda-lime absorber.
Arrows indicate gas pathways.
From Whitten and Wise (10); *courtesy: British Journal of Anaesthesia*

and the breathing bag collapses. Flushing with oxygen has led at least once to a
tension pneumothorax, but the mere exclusion of the pressure relief valve in this
event is of sufficient import to warrant the condemnation of this arrangement.

A probably unique accident has been described by Edwards and associates
(3). An absorber fell off a machine while the patient was paralyzed. Ventilation
could not be re-instituted in time and the patient died.

The following case from our own departmental files illustrates another potential hazard following preventive maintenance:

*A pneumothorax developed in a 49-year-old male who underwent an operation
for duodenal ulcer. As soon as the patient had been connected to the anaesthetic
machine after tracheal intubation, it was noted that the breathing bag was not
inflating properly on exhalation. On examining the machine, it was seen that a
bushing in the 'on-off' control of a Heidbrink circle absorber had been replaced
in the reversed position, thus blocking deflation of the lung.*

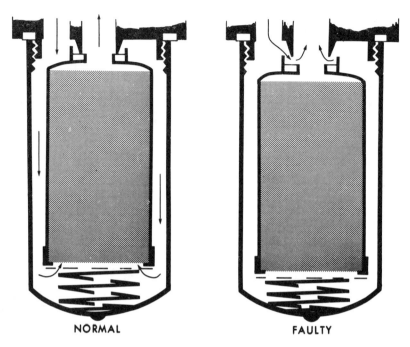

Figure 24 / Normal and faulty condition of BOC Boyle Mark 2 soda-lime absorber. Arrows indicate gas pathways.
From Whitten and Wise (10); *courtesy: British Journal of Anaesthesia*

Ringrose (9) and others (4, 5) have drawn attention to a design characteristic of the Mark III Boyle circle absorber in which the corrugated hose from the reservoir bag and that forming the expiratory limb of the circle not only join in close proximity but also are connected to the absorber by male fittings of identical diameter. If erroneous interchange of the two hoses is made, immediate high pressures accumulate within the inspiratory limb and, in the case described, led to bilateral pneumothorax. The design of the Boyle absorber has been changed in subsequent models to reduce the chance of such errors.

Whitten and Wise (10) have drawn attention to other design faults in absorbers. In the case of the MIE Lincoln 800 soda-lime absorber, the fault lies in the fact that the inner soda-lime carrier may cease to be properly supported so that it assumes a lower position within its housing. This opens an avenue for the escape of gases before they pass through the soda-lime. Since the entire assembly is transparent, it should be possible to detect the fault by inspection (Fig. 23). In the case of the BOC Boyle Mark II absorber, a similar situation can arise (Fig. 24).

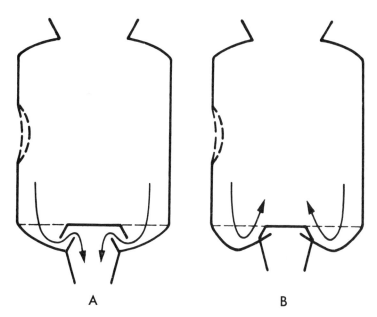

Figure 25 / A, normal absorber; B, bent base. Arrows indicate gas pathways. *From Beyermann-Urbig* (1); *courtesy: Der Anaesthesist*

In this instance the leak may be caused by weakening of the spring in the base of the outer carrier, or by the fact that the dimensions of canister and carrier vary slightly from model to model so that one canister may function efficiently in one apparatus but not in another.

That equipment on which the life of the patient may depend must be treated with care and consideration is emphasized by the experience of Beyermann-Urbig (1) who found that the base of their absorber had been bent from an externally convex to a concave configuration, thus almost entirely obstructing the gas exit (Fig. 25). While there was no difficulty inflating the lungs, deflation was difficult and incomplete.

Although now used infrequently, some remarks concerning the Waters' to-and-fro canister should be made. Difficulties with this item often are related to its vicinity to the patient's face. Heat retention is a definite danger unless canisters are changed frequently, as are inhalation of dust, or caustic liquid reaching the patient if the absorbent becomes too wet. Leaks are common because contact is difficult to maintain because of the weight of the poorly supported heavy canister, or as a result of having been dropped on the floor. Deadspace increases as the absorbent becomes used up.

As with all canisters, to-and-fro or circle, proper packing of contents is essential or channelling of gases will occur, with loss of absorption efficiency and increase of deadspace.

VALVES

Most anaesthetic systems incorporate one or more valves in the breathing system to direct gas flow or to facilitate exit of gases from the system. Common to all is the danger that they may stick or fail to close.

A case has been described of complete respiratory obstruction whenever the mask was applied to the patient's face (1). On testing the machine the breathing bag did not empty when the mask was removed from the patient's face while the expiratory valve was closed. On further inspection, it was found that the rubber leaflet of the inspiratory valve was firmly stuck to the valve seat so that gas flow to the patient was completely blocked.

One of the most common and most hazardous situations created solely by valves is related to the use of the valved Y-piece (Fig. 26A, B). This particular item of equipment was introduced originally to reduce deadspace in a circle system. Theoretically this appeared to be an excellent solution, but it has become obvious that the use of this type of Y-piece introduced potential hazards into the practice of anaesthesia which far outweighed its advantages. Since carbon dioxide absorbers are provided with a set of undirectional valves of their own, one on the inspiratory and one on the expiratory side, it follows that unless the valve leaflets are removed from the absorber, the use of the valved Y-piece introduces a second set of valves into the system. No harm results from this unless the Y-piece has been connected with valves in opposition to the direction of gas flow imparted by the valves on the absorber. Should this occur, no gas can flow to the patient, but pressure increases on the inflow side of the circle since gas entering the inspiratory corrugated tubing is held up by the valve in the Y-piece and cannot return because of the competent inspiratory valve on the absorber. Over the entire time the patient's lungs are not being ventilated. As there is no return flow of gases, the breathing bag is collapsed if it is on the expiratory side of the circle, or it can be filled but not emptied if it is on the inspiratory side (13). As a consequence either the inspiratory breathing tube ruptures or the corresponding valve in the Y-piece does, allowing gas to enter the trachea at the high accumulated pressure (2) (Fig. 27). In one such case (8), because the breathing bag was not filling, the system was flushed several times with oxygen, which caused the valve on the inspiratory side of the Y-piece to buckle with consequent development of wide-spread subcutaneous emphysema, tension pneumothorax, pneumomediastinum, and pneumoperitoneum.

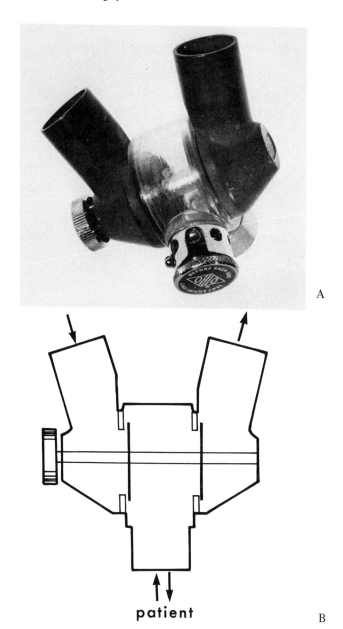

Figure 26 / A, The valved Y-piece. B, The valved Y-piece (cross section).

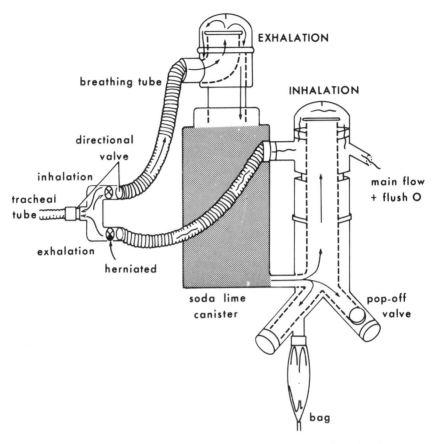

Figure 27 / Schematic representation of gas flow in a circuit with valved Y-piece and opposed valves.
From Doǧu and Davis (8); courtesy: Anesthesiology

Conversely, if the valve leaflets have been removed from the absorber because the valved Y-piece has been used and are not replaced at the end of the operation and if, during subsequent use, an ordinary non-valved Y-piece is substituted, the system will be devoid of any valves whatsoever, in which case the gas flow in the circle is not being directed at all and the entire circle system is converted to deadspace. We, in common with other departments, have such a case on record. Of course, accidents of this kind can be avoided entirely if valves are checked before the machine is put into use (7). A similar situation arises if the valves become incompetent. This may be due to repeated autoclaving of the valved

Y-piece with consequent distortion of the leaflets, valve seats, or both (10). White (18) reports that during one single conversation with fellow anaesthetists he was appraised of no less than three incidents of difficulties arising out of the use of valved funnel Y-pieces. It is because of the number of serious accidents reported with this type of equipment that the ASA Sub-committee on Standardization has recommended that valved Y-pieces not be used (19). Nevertheless they are still in isolated use to wreak havoc, as evidenced by a recent inquest (3).

Another valve which has been giving trouble from time to time is the *Ruben non-rebreathing valve*. Effective function of this valve depends upon the pressure drop at the inlet. If re-breathing occurs, it can lead not only to hypercarbia but under some circumstances to overdosage with inhalation anaesthetics as well (5). Askrog and Elb (4) have demonstrated that when blow-through bags are used with this type of valve, outside pressure is exerted on the bag. This causes the valve to open and considerable spill of gas occurs as shown by elevation of alveolar carbon dioxide. Such a situation does not occur with the Magill system even if manual ventilation is used, likely because the bag is hanging free. Askrog and Elb as well as Vogel, Hakim, and Pflüger (17) have shown that great differences exist between one valve and another in terms of re-breathing due to the delay of the valve at the end of expiration which has a tendency to remain in the inspiratory position. Reduction in the size of the valve disk will eliminate this cause of re-breathing. Meyer (11) has reported that with both new and old Ruben valves, be it during spontaneous or positive pressure breathing, leaks occur which result in a mixture of room air with fresh gas, re-breathing of carbon dioxide containing gas, and leakage of fresh gas into the environment during positive pressure inspiration. These assertions have been strongly contested by Ruben himself (14) who has contended that these findings are of no practical significance because investigations were made with a mechanical ventilator unsuitable for this purpose. In the absence of conclusive measurements supporting one or the other position, the performance of this valve must remain under suspicion. Holland (9) has described two fatalities due to accidental jamming of Ruben non-rebreathing valves in the inspiratory position. This caused catastrophic interpulmonary pressures because gas could not escape.

When using the *Stephen-Slater non-rebreathing valve* one should be aware of a unique potential difficulty inherent in the construction of this device. The assembly consists of two flutter valves, one external expiratory and one internal inspiratory mounted on a cylinder which fits snugly within the metal housing of the valve. The cylinder can become displaced towards the patient end of the valve (Fig. 28), partially or even completely occluding the expiratory valve. Exhalation then becomes impeded or totally obstructed. In one of our own cases the cylinder had been moved all the way into the patient side of the valve

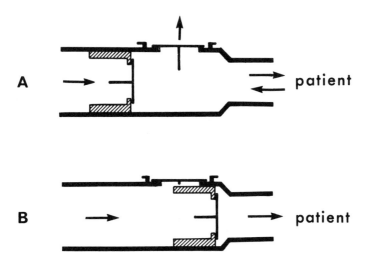

Figure 28 / Schematic cross section of Stephen-Slater non-rebreathing valve.
A, Normal. B, Cylinder carrying the inspiratory valve displaced and occluding
the expiratory port.

housing, thus placing the exhalation valve behind the inhalation one and blocking gas flow from the patient completely.

Difficulties with other valve systems have been relatively uncommon. The
widely used one-way disc valves in circle systems are remarkably reliable, provided the disc is in place. Although they have a glass cover to facilitate inspection of the discs, it is not always easy to see if they have been replaced after
servicing. Dean, Parsons, and Raphaely (6) have reported a case of bilateral
pneumothorax due to a displaced flutter valve of an Ohio absorber (Fig. 29). It
is assumed in this case that during cleaning the valve on the absorber had fallen
accidentally between the inner and outer casings of the expiratory valve housing
and had ultimately migrated to a position directly above the inlet for the reservoir bag. In doing so it allowed gas to enter the system but not to exit, leading to
an accumulation of pressure. In a communication from Australia, Russell and Drew
(15) point out that one of two types of inspiratory valves in the circle system of the
CIG Medishield Boyle machine may be fitted. In the preferred configuration the
fresh gas inlet enters the inner chamber on the absorber side, upstream of the valve.
In the other, the fresh gas inlet is fixed to the wall of the inner chamber, but does
not communicate with it. Fresh gas enters the outer chamber through a hole on the
underside of the fresh gas tube. Both types of valves are identically labelled and
cannot be distinguished by external inspection. This represents a potential hazard.

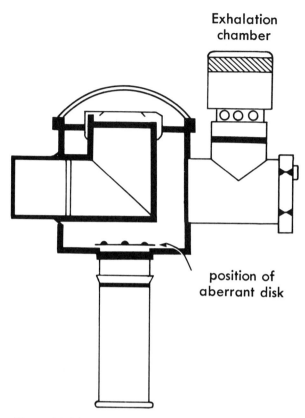

Exhalation chamber

position of aberrant disk

Figure 29 / Schematic representation of expiratory chamber of anaesthesia machine with disc in aberrent position above the pipe leading to the reservoir bag.
From Dean, Parsons, and Raphaely (6); courtesy: Anesthesia and Analgesia — Current Researches

Records from our department yield yet another case of difficulties with valves:

A 42-year-old woman received a general anaesthetic and full curarization with tracheal intubation. Immediately upon being connected to the circle circuit, it was noticed that the breathing bag did not move on exhalation. Each time the bag was compressed, inspiratory chest movements were produced but no deflation followed. The circle absorber system was immediately disconnected, and a

Magill attachment was substituted. This resulted in respiratory exchange with controlled respiration. On examination of the circle system it was found that the absorber carried two inlet valves but no expiratory valve, the wrong replacement valve having been supplied by the manufacturer.

Holland (9) has recommended that a pressure-limiting safety device should always be interposed between any non-rebreathing valve and the patient. Any ordinary expiratory relief valve could serve this purpose well. In order to avoid hazards connected with the development of dangerously high pressures in any breathing circuit, Norry (12) and also Rasz and Duncalf (16) have described pressure-limiting valves which can be adapted to any anaesthetic machine. While it would appear advisable to incorporate such valves as standard equipment into anaesthesia circuits, the development of excessive pressure in the breathing system can be avoided by prescribing that a suitably compliant reservoir bag be always in the system.

CONNECTORS AND ADAPTORS

The International Standards Organization draft on anaesthetic nomenclature defines connectors as fittings intended to join together two or more components, while adaptors establish functional continuity between otherwise disparate or incompatible components. Thus they are specialized connectors. Although in a strict sense they are 'adaptors' by these definitions, we shall follow established practice and refer here to 'tracheal tube connectors.' In the United States, connection is made by the direct mating of male and female joints of standard diameter and taper (Fig. 30A), while in the British usage a catheter mount of rubber or other flexible material serves as a bridge between two rigid components, the opposing ends of which then no longer need to be of standard size and configuration (Fig. 30B).

The American tracheal tube connector may be straight or curved. If straight, a curved intermediate connector often is placed between it and the patient end of the breathing tube. This connector may or may not have a limb or 'chimney' intended to accommodate a tracheal suction catheter. The common British connector is curved or right-angled, a common prototype being the Cobb suction union or Rowbotham connector (Fig. 31).

Connectors, of whatever kind, must fit snugly into their respective tracheal tubes so that they may not become detached. The following case from our files is only one example of the seriousness of this particular accident:

A 40-year-old big muscular man was anaesthetized for tonsillectomy. Tracheal intubation was difficult even after relatively large amounts of muscle relaxant

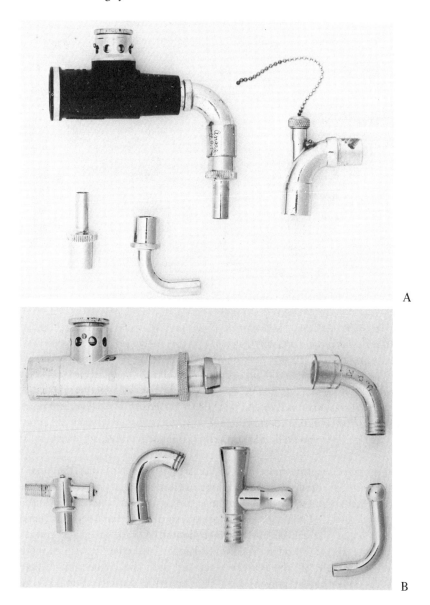

A

B

Figure 30 / Pressure relief valve and various connectors: A, direct connection —
American usage; B, indirect connection — British usage.

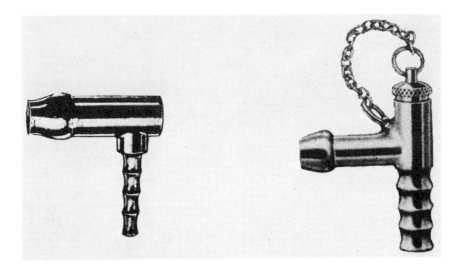

Figure 31 / *Left*, Rowbotham connector; *right*, Cobb suction union.

because of a thick neck and small mouth. Eventually the tube was passed but because of a fleshy tongue and difficulty in opening his mouth, the surgeon had trouble inserting the mouth gag. Eventually he succeeded, but in doing so the tracheal tube became detached from its connector and sprang back into the nasopharynx. Considerable difficulty was experienced in removing the tube, again because of the small mouth and because of the position in which the tube had settled itself. The patient became deeply cyanosed, but eventually the tube was recovered and reconnected, and the patient did not come to any harm.

Furthermore connectors must not be so large in diameter that the tube is stretched over them, predisposing to kinking just distal to the patient end of the connector. Where connections without intervening catheter mounts are used, care must be taken that they are not deformed, so that the bond remains secure and without leaks, yet can be broken when desired. Nevertheless such connections can come apart, although this should happen infrequently with properly maintained equipment of the correct taper and with the connection initially firmly made. However to prevent such an occurrence entirely, Star (19) has recommended that an L-shaped slit be made into the distal portion of the Y-piece to receive a small tip welded to the metal connector of the tracheal tube. This will result in a bayonet joint which will prevent disengagement of the connector from the Y-piece. Dolan (4) has described a spiral bayonet connector which ensures seal of the taper cone and compensates for wear. This is considered more satisfactory than the straight bayonet described by Star.

Right-angled connectors are manufactured by joining together two distinct metal parts and therefore, if a side opening has not been made in the vertical limb before the horizontal one is joined to it, an imperforate device results. This leads immediately to total respiratory obstruction as soon as the device has been attached to the breathing circuit. Such occurrences, although infrequent, have been described for both the Cobb and the Rowbotham units (5, 15). Total obstruction also has occurred in a straight plastic tracheal tube connector which was found to have a membrane across its lumen (13). Still another cause of obstruction of a connector has been described where its outside was lubricated before insertion into the machine end of the tracheal tube. The lubricating jelly then found its way into the inside of the connector where it dried and eventually formed a solid plug (12). If drying is slow, a hollow cylinder with a central film may form which, in turn, may then break down, leading to narrowing of the lumen rather than complete obstruction. In another instance described by Hewer (8) a bakelite spigot normally used to close the inflating tube on the pneumatic cushion of a face mask became wedged in the Cobb suction union, the shoulder of the spigot acting as a non-return valve, while in Stark's case (20) the offender was a spare 'one-way' inflating valve for the cuff which blocked his 15-mm tracheal tube connector and in Collier's case it was the plastic screw cap from a winged infusion set (3).

In another case reported by Shaw (17) it was found impossible to ventilate the lungs after tracheal intubation. The trachea was re-intubated and when no cause was found in the discarded tracheal tube, the adaptor was bivalved for closer examination. Only then a large plug of hardened PVC was noted. This probably had become lodged there prior to autoclaving, had melted, and then re-hardened into a solid mass. The presence of a dead cockroach within the lumen of a Cobb connection is somewhat less easily explained (18). McKinley (11) encountered a connector which was totally occluded by a thin, almost invisible plastic membrane just inside the patient end. This connector had been packaged on cardboard under a clear plastic film applied by heat under a vacuum. In the course of this process the plastic material had come to be drawn into the connector and had remained there when the connector was removed from the package.

Obstruction of Cobb suction unions has come about in yet another fashion. These units are marketed by different manufacturers, the vertical limb above the right angle on the BOC adaptor being longer than that of the MIE device (Fig. 32A). If the rubber plug destined to occlude the vertical suction limb on the BOC connector is inserted into the shorter MIE limb, it may then be so long as to reach beyond the right-angle portion, with the result that gas flow from the

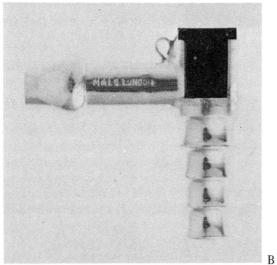

A

B

Figure 32 / A, Two types of Cobb suction unions; *left*, BOC model;
right, MIE variety. B, The long BOC plug has been inserted into the short
BOC suction limb of a Cobb suction union, completely obstructing the gas flow.
From Ross (16); *courtesy: Anaesthesia*

horizontal limb may be obstructed where it joins the vertical limb (16) (Fig. 32B). Consequently, it is advisable that only one type of connector should be available in any one department to obviate at least this one hazard. Also, if caps were used instead of plugs, one potential source of difficulties would be avoided. Haley (7) has described a similar situation in which the fresh gas inflow into a 'Montreal' Pediatric circuit became obstructed because of the interposition of a plastic right-angled connector between the T-piece and the straight tracheal tube connector. The plastic angle fitted so deeply into the T-piece that it occluded its inflow limb (Fig. 33). Accidents of this kind can be avoided by using only equipment of standard dimensions in which the taper of the male portion will prevent unduly deep penetration. To guard further against wear of the taper which can occur with hard-rubber appliances, a stop could be provided which might consist of a pin or the inflow limb itself protruding into the lumen of the T-piece or a shoulder on the male connector.

The catheter mount on the other hand, because of its non-rigid construction, may by its very nature kink, bend, or twist, especially if it is too long (1). In order to avoid this complication the mount should just bridge the gap between the metal parts, which may even be in contact with one another. Also non-kinkable mounts have been employed with advantage. They may be of similar construction as corrugated breathing tubes or they may consist of metal or nylon coils embedded in latex or other anti-static material. The latter type of mount is manufactured by a process of repeated dipping so that several layers of material are formed around the spiral base. The innermost of these layers may become detached with the insertion of the tracheal tube connector which may cause it to invaginate or pucker, resulting in partial or complete airway obstruction (2, 9, 10, 14). Problems arising out of the layering in reinforced tubes will be discussed in more detail in the chapter dealing with non-kinkable tracheal tubes.

Improvisations involving the joining together of pieces which do not mate are particularly dangerous and certainly should not become part of routine procedure. The following case is an illustration of the difficulties which can arise when this principle is ignored:

A 55-year-old man was anaesthetized for repair of a compound fracture of the temporal bone. Tracheal intubation was difficult and the larynx could not be visualized. Whenever the tube was felt to be in the trachea, ventilation was impossible, so that the tube had to be withdrawn and again re-inserted. Eventually mouth-to-tube respiration was tried and this was successful. Inspection of the catheter mount now revealed that it was plugged, although it had been patent during an earlier operation. This catheter mount consisted of two non-fitting

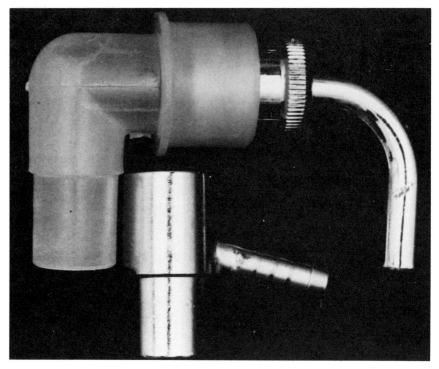

Figure 33 / The plastic right-angled connector, when inserted into the T-piece, will obstruct the inflow limb because of its length.
From: Haley (7); courtesy: Canadian Anaesthetists' Society Journal

metal portions joined by adhesive tape and encased in a plastic sheath. Rotation of the metal pieces around the longitudinal axis had twisted the adhesive tape like the diaphragm of a camera so that the lumen had become occluded.

Equipment of this nature should, of course, never be used or, if assembled as a temporary makeshift, should be disassembled and discarded immediately after use.

We had occasion to refer to the presence of foreign materials within parts of the anaesthetic machine (p. 23). Particles can also derive from plating of the inside of metal connectors and are equally hazardous, especially in view of the fact that they are even closer to the patient's airway than those occurring within the machine. We have found such metal chips in a flexible connector (Fig. 34)

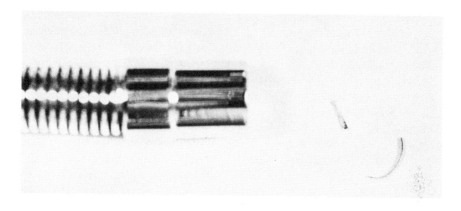

Figure 34 / Flexible metal connector with metal chips recovered from its lumen.

and one must again emphasize that it is undesirable to have plating on the inside of any metal parts of the breathing circuit. Galway (6) found a piece of macerated absorbent paper towel partially occluding the lumen of a catheter mount. This probably remained as the result of an attempt to dry the inside of the mount after immersion in an antiseptic solution.

SCAVENGING DEVICES*

The possible association between chronic exposure to anaesthetic gases and disease states in operating room personnel is at the moment largely based on circumstantial evidence (8, 9, 22), but cannot be ignored. Nor can the possible effects of anaesthetic gases on perceptual, cognitive, and motor skills be disregarded (3, 4). The result has been the production of a series of devices for the removal of waste anaesthetic gases, beginning with simple adaptations of existing equipment (1, 2, 6, 11, 12, 13, 15, 17, 20, 21, 23, 24).

Some of these devices were developed commercially, and derivatives of them are now being widely used. Development is as yet by no means complete, and a new generation of more sophisticated devices is just starting to be marketed.

The methods of scavenging can be divided into three main groups, each with its own hazards: (1) operating room ventilation, (2) passive systems, (3) powered systems.

* This section has been contributed by Dr J.K. Scott.

Operating room ventilation
The use of ventilation alone as a means of rapidly removing inhalational anaesthetic gases from the operating room is impractical because of the engineering
problems involved, the cost, and the unpleasant environment that extremely
rapid air changes would create. However, ventilation is used in conjunction with
either passive or powered systems, provided it is of the non-recirculating kind.

Many anaesthetists and hospital engineers are unaware of the actual air flow
patterns in their own operating rooms, and this is borne out by past experience
both in our department and elsewhere (7). In three of our theatres we found
that exhaust grills were non-functional, and that under certain circumstances,
one actually could act as an air inlet. Prior investigation of exhaust grills is,
therefore, essential if their use for venting of anaesthetic gases is contemplated.
Some ventilation systems have dual modes of operation and may be set to
recirculate, and when so set, must not be used for venting.

Passive systems
Passive systems were first developed as a means of conducting explosive anaesthetic gas mixtures away from the operating room (5). Originally devised with
T-piece junctions, and now utilizing a variety of shrouded valves or T-pieces, the
passive system utilizes the elastic recoil of the lungs to expel waste gas down a
tube which is vented.

The most obvious factor to the observing anaesthetist is the loss of the valve
noise in a spontaneously breathing, or ventilated patient. Many anaesthetists rely
on these auditory signals as a monitor of respiration.

The length of the venting tubing, its diameter, and its construction are important. The resistance along a tube varies according to its length, its diameter, and
the number of bends in it. Too high a resistance in a passive venting tube may
produce positive end-expiratory pressure on the breathing system.

Obstruction of the venting tubing, unless fitted with a pressure releasing
interface will result in increased pressure within the breathing system (p. 93)
(10). Interfaces to cope with passive scavenging and provide pressure relief are
available, but some are attached to the anaesthetic machine, leaving a length of
tube between the interface and the expiratory valve which can become obstructed. The position of the interface is critical and should be on, or as near
as possible to the expiratory valve.

The size of tubing involved in scavenging devices should be different in size
from any other tubing used in the anaesthetic circuit, with different sized connectors to eliminate the possibility of misconnections. Although manufacturers
are reluctant to utilize tubing other than conductive rubber or neoprene, a good
case can be made for the utilization of light-weight smooth conductive plastic

tubing for the scavenging systems which could even be coloured to distinguish it from the patient circuit. The current sizes in most common use at present are 30 mm, 19 mm, and 18 mm tubing, but no agreement as to a universal standard size appears in sight.

Condensation of water vapour within a passive system may result in obstruction or act as a medium for bacterial growth and contamination. Therefore passive systems should incorporate some form of water trap to eliminate this problem.

The dumping site of the anaesthetic gases is also important. Two main sites are used: the operating room exhaust grill or the outside atmosphere.

If vented into the hospital exhaust system, the eventual dumping site should be investigated to make sure that the waste gases are not sucked into another part of the hospital. The gases must be able to disperse rapidly in the atmosphere without causing further contamination. The type of fan used to drive the exhaust system is also important, since it is known that halothane causes degradation of oil in pumps and bearings (16). If externally vented, the outlet must be protected against pressure variations due to wind, and the entry of dust, insects, and rodents. Several centimeters of positive or negative water pressure can be generated in passive ducting as a result of variations in external ambient pressures, and valve systems to prevent this add to the overall resistance in the system.

A variation on the passive system is the filtering of waste gases, vented passively through activated charcoal (23). This has the disadvantage of selective adsorption and in particular poor removal of nitrous oxide. Some adsorbers constitute a fire-hazard since they consist of an enhanced concentration of oxygen and nitrous oxide with finely divided charcoal in a cardboard and nonconducting plastic case (16).

Powered scavenging
The unavailability of suitable theatre exhaust, or the cost of constructing passive venting systems has resulted in widespread use of suction devices powered by a variety of means to remove waste gases. The most convenient pathway is the hospital vacuum system. It is simple to install and free from the problems of retrograde flows and uncontrolled disposal. However NFPA regulations in the United States and Canadian regulations forbid the disposal of flammable gases into central vacuum systems.

In all these devices suction is applied to a reservoir into which the patient's expired gases flow passively, and are mixed with entrained air.

In the designs currently available the reservoir size varies considerably and so do the flow rates. The simpler devices have restricted suction orifices, whereas more sophisticated models have flow-regulating devices. In most large hospitals flow through a particular vacuum unit varies according to demand on the system. In tests in our department (18) there was approximately a 30 per cent drop in flow through any one unit, when all the other vacuum units in the operating room suite were turned on. In a fixed orifice device, such a drop in flow may well allow the escape of waste gases through the air entraining orifice.

The most dangerous hazard is, of course, the risk of pulmonary barotrauma should a high negative pressure be applied to the system causing a malfunction of the expiratory valve (19). This can easily occur if the entraining orifice is occluded, and usually these are close to the floor, near drapes, etc. which may be sucked over the orifice. A negative pressure relief valve should be *mandatory* to prevent this hazard in all powered devices utilizing negative pressure. A positive pressure interface device should also be considered because of the risk of development of a high pressure in the breathing system for similar reasons to those advocated for the passive circuit.

The ideal system of powered evacuation should have its own pump, whether this be in each operating room or removed from it and possibly serving more than one room. The problems with individual pumps are that they are noisy and that, if any leakage should occur before the gases are dumped, the system, being positively pressurized, will tend to release its contents to the atmosphere in the operating room.

Finally a word about the efficiency of the various scavengers and scavenging systems. Scavenging devices vary in their efficiency and a few systems were not designed to cope with the variations in a variety of conditions possible in clinical practice and may allow the escape of pollutants. All systems must be evaluated under the conditions in which they are to be used, employing suitable testing apparatus.

Previous experience with scavenging, both in our unit and elsewhere (14) shows that equipment requires constant supervision, monitoring, and service, since very slight leaks, especially in high pressure lines and circuits, can produce significant pollution.

V
Accessories to the anaesthetic machine and special equipment

Ventilators are the most complicated mechanical equipment used by anaesthetists and are certainly the most diverse. There are innumerable models available of both the pressure cycled and volume cycled varieties, driven by gas or electricity and based on a number of different mechanical principles. Any one of these ventilators may malfunction at any time but, given their great diversity, it is difficult if not impossible to extrapolate from a misadventure with one particular apparatus to another, or to consider all failures theoretically possible in each of the many varied kinds of apparatus. Since there is such a variety of ventilators, it is the more surprising to find a remarkable paucity of reports of malfunctions in the literature. As patients unable to breathe on their own are dependent upon ventilators for their very existence, one can only surmise that the limited number of reports of misadventures must be based on fear of litigation. Nevertheless, an attempt can and should be made to classify malfunctions and three broad common denominators can be identified with relative ease; one group comprises cases of inadequate ventilation, one of overdistension of the lungs, and one of the unintentional entrainment of air.

Inadequate ventilation
Inadequate ventilation may be of varying degrees and is not necessarily due to malfunction of equipment. In the extreme it may reach the point where no movement of gas takes place into and out of the lungs. Obviously, when this happens, immediate remedial action must be taken, preferably by disconnecting the patient from the ventilator and instituting manual lung ventilation with an Ambu bag, anaesthetic machine, or similar device capable of inflating the lungs, while the mechanical malfunction of the ventilator is being corrected or a

substitute ventilator is being procured. If the ventilator has merely become disconnected from the patient, immediate reconnection or substitution by manual or mouth-to-tube ventilation is, of course, mandatory. Since disconnection is the commonest cause of ventilator failure, it follows that patients on mechanical ventilation must be observed continuously. This is a particularly onerous assignment since difficulties arise suddenly without warning often after long periods of uneventful ventilation, a situation which predisposes to slack minute-to-minute observation and demands a high degree of concentration. Many patients indeed have lost their lives for just that reason. A number of ISO sub-committees are addressing themselves to this very urgent problem, with a view to reducing, if not eliminating, the incidence of these tragic events. Overton and Miceli (18) have designed a disconnection alarm for the Bennett BA-4 ventilator which will operate when the ventilator is pressure limited. Unfortunately, alarms in general are not one hundred per cent reliable, may be switched off, or may be ignored because of habituation to false alarms.

Simionescu (22) has described a case where the *East-Radcliffe* ventilator failed to deliver any gas, while the pressure gauge still recorded normal inflation pressures. The reason for this was that the valve at the base of the bellows which provides the positive pressure had jammed in the open position. As a result, gas flowed back into the reservoir bag instead of into the anaesthetic circuit, so that no flow resulted. The valve was stuck to the cage assembly because it had become soiled by the melted seal of the rubber seating at the base of the assembly. This points to the important requirement that valves be visible, a requirement not met by many ventilators and one of the reasons for many undetected malfunctions. The Bennett monitoring spirometer has similarly been known to indicate ventilation when in fact no fresh gases reached the patient's lungs (see below). Of course, harm will only result if undue reliance is placed on such mechanical devices at the expense of diligent observation of the patient.

It has been reported that a number of *Bennett MA-1 volume* ventilators equipped with the Puritan Bennett optional Flow Rate Circuit Cards have unpredictably stopped, failed to start, or have spontaneously changed their cycling rate. The source of the defect has been located and the necessary corrections are being made by the manufacturers. Rectifier failure in the power supply of a few *Siemens-Elema Servo* ventilators 900 has caused loss of respiratory support (4), and although this particular model is no longer being sold, these occurrences nevertheless point again to the necessity of continuous observation of patients on ventilators and the immediate availability of alternate means to ventilate the lungs should the mechanical ventilator fail (2).

The *Bennett Monitoring Spirometer* which is used on Bennett and other ventilators can appear to indicate ventilation when the expiratory valve diaphragm or its tubing has failed and the patient's lungs in actual fact are not being ventilated (1). To complicate matters it has been found that the alarm which is an option with this spirometer may not be activated in some instances of this kind of failure. Figure 35 shows schematically the principle of this spirometer. During inspiratory flow the gas inflates the diaphragm to seal the expiratory port and direct the flow to the patient. During the expiratory phase the diaphragm empties with the result that the exhalation port opens and the patient is allowed to exhale passively into the spirometer. If the expiratory valve diaphragm fails or if its tubing becomes disconnected, most or all of the expiratory flow escapes direct into the spirometer, bypassing the patient. The spirometer under these circumstances fills during inspiration rather than expiration. Whether the alarm becomes activated or not will depend on whether the volume filling the spirometer is greater or less than that set to activate the alarm. This volume will to a large extent depend upon the ventilator used. There have been instances in which the spirometer has continued to fill to approximately the normal volume after the expiratory valve has become disconnected, but no alarm sounded even though the patient's lungs were not being ventilated.

Desautels and Modell (9) have recommended the insertion of a modified Stephen-Slater non-rebreathing valve into the inspiratory limb of volume-cycled ventilators which function as closed units, so that complete airway obstruction does not result should malfunction occur since air can be entrained into the system.

Less severe hypoventilation, short of total or near-total non-ventilation, may come about through leaks in the system. Leaks in ventilators are rare when compared with those from other parts of the gas flow sequence; nevertheless, the possibility must be borne in mind when abnormally high gas flows are needed and all other sources of leaks have been excluded. Rolbin (19) for instance reports one case, and refers to another similar one, in which the leak was traced to damage of the metal connecting pipe which serves the additional purpose of supporting the *Air Shields Ventimeter* ventilator.

Overinflation

The second category of malfunctions relates to overinflation of the lungs. This is a very real danger and indeed many of the published cases relate to just that particular hazard. Most often this kind of accident is related to impediment of gas return from the lungs. This can occur for a variety of reasons. For instance, Gamble and Coppel (13) point out that with the variable orifice type of expiratory 'retard' there is a danger of producing very high airway pressures if a large expiratory flow is produced against the considerable resistance of the retard as with coughing, for instance. High pressures are less likely to occur when springloaded valves are used as retards, unless the valve, being unidirectional, is inserted the wrong way round, in which case it will block exhalation completely.

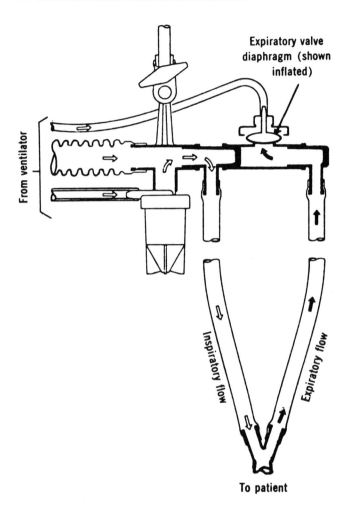

Figure 35 / The Bennett monitoring spirometer. White arrows indicate the inspiratory flow which also serves to inflate the expiratory valve thus occluding the expiratory flow (solid arrows).
Courtesy: Health Devices (1)

They recommend that where valves of this type are used the inspiratory and expiratory sides should be made non-interchangeable. Another solution could be to design a valve with two diaphragms and springs in parallel, each allowing flow in a direction opposite to the other. Thus one or the other valve will be operative in whichever direction it is inserted.

Arkinstall and Epstein (5) reported the occurrence of a bilateral pneumo-thorax after a *Bird Mark VIII* ventilator failed to cycle and consequently the patient's lungs were exposed to continuous positive pressure. In this particular case the connecting shaft running through the ceramic valve had broken, thus permitting the machine to continue in the pressure cycle.

The *Bird Mark IV*, used in conjunction with an anaesthetic machine, has two openings on its side, one to take the breathing hose and the other for attachment of the breathing bag for manual ventilation. Spoerel (23) has pointed out that, although the two openings are appropriately marked, the attachments are inter-changeable. If an error is made and the bag and breathing hose are interchanged, the attachment leading to the patient is closed off. Since exits from the breath-ing system usually are closed when the patient is placed on the ventilator, no outlet exists for the gas reaching the patient direct from the anaesthetic machine and pressure will build up rapidly. Non-interchangeability of these two openings is desirable.

In 1965 Morrow and associates (17) described a tension pneumothorax result-ing from erroneous connection of a *'Ventimeter'* ventilator. Here the corrugated tubing from the circle system had been connected to the ventilator fitting de-signed to hold the reservoir bag, while the bag in turn was attached to the fitting for the tubing. In this configuration the bellows of the ventilator will not fill. If either the bag fill valve on the ventilator or the oxygen flush valve on the anaesthetic machine is activated, the pressure in the breathing system will in-crease rapidly to dangerous levels and this may lead to a tension pneumothorax and/or circulatory collapse. To prevent future mishaps of this kind the authors have had the bag connection enlarged so that its diameter is larger than the internal diameter of the tubing used to connect to the breathing circuit. Unfor-tunately, this enlarged bag fitting is just the right diameter to hold the metal pipe which in many departments supports the ventilator. Consequently, it has been advised that a pin be inserted through the bag fitting to prevent any interchange of this kind–a situation that has occurred (10). Despite all these precautions, Turndorf, Capan, and Kessel (24) had an experience similar to Morrow's nine years later, and even more recently Sears and Bocar (20) have encountered it again in a *Monaghan 300* ventilator.

Accidental closure of the expiratory outlet in an *Engström* ventilator by the metal cork which seals the water humidifier has been reported by Sia (21). During automatic ventilation the flow of gas in this case is first directed to the water humidifier expiratory limb tubing, then to the patient end, then to the inspiratory limb tubing, and back to the humidifier. There is, therefore, no exit of gas and as a result high pressure may develop in the system. It is recom-mended that the metal cork for the humidifier outlet be made non-interchange-able with the other inlet and outlet ports of the ventilator.

In another example the expiratory hose on a *Cape* ventilator cabinet was disconnected from its port in order to drain condensed water. On reconnection it was mistakenly attached to the patient air intake valve rather than to its own port, with the result that expiration could not occur while inspiration continued (26). Here too the solution was to weld a bar across the air intake, making it impossible to insert the expiratory hose into this particular port. The sudden occurrence of tension pneumothorax is a possibility that must always be kept in mind when patients are on ventilators. This misadventure can occur suddenly even after many days and weeks of uneventful mechanical ventilation and if not immediately recognized can be quickly fatal. Such a case happened in our intensive care unit some months ago in the middle of the night.

Entrainment of air or oxygen

This is the third major group of malfunctions. It involves the danger of awareness during maintenance of anaesthesia and has been referred to by Waters (25) in the context of a discussion of factors causing awareness during operations.

The *Cape Waine* ventilator has a negative pressure limiting valve which should open at −15 cm water but on the particular ventilator described by Bookallil (7) it opened at −4 cm. As a result air was being entrained into the system. This is a difficult defect to detect and in this case it took 18 months and several instances of awareness before the cause was recognized. Hurdley (14) has drawn attention to a hazard in the *East Radcliffe* ventilator which can arise if the air intake fitting is rotated counter-clockwise. Such rotation can occur if the absorption cannister is repeatedly attached and removed. The ventilator is fitted with a spring-loaded air inlet valve which is incorporated as a safety measure so that air may be entrained if gases are not flowing or if they are insufficient for patient requirement. The rotation of the air intake fitting causes depression of the bracket which supports the breathing tube, and the pressure exerted by the bracket holds the valve fully open. If this occurs, the anaesthetic gases will be diluted to the point where anaesthesia may become inadequate. A modification of the valve cap has been designed to control this particular difficulty (12).

A case of entrainment which occurred in our department is relevant in this connection:

A 47-year-old patient was to undergo anterior cervical fusion for cervical spondylosis. Anaesthesia was with nitrous oxide and azeotrope halothane-ether following induction with thiopentone. A Bird Mark IV ventilator was used with a gas flow of three litres of nitrous oxide and one litre of oxygen in a circle absorber circuit. The anaesthetic proceeded uneventfully, but when the patient was seen on the afternoon after the operation she related that she remembered certain events during the operation, that she had drifted in and out of anaesthesia but when awake had also felt pain. In view of the fact that a volatile anaesthetic had been added to the nitrous oxide-oxygen mixture, it was obvious that air or oxygen must have been entrained somewhere along the respiratory circuit and it was then ascertained that this had indeed happened in that the tidal volume lever had been set in such a way as to allow the bellows to activate the emergency fill.

Miscellaneous observations

Accuracy of ventilators is a matter of concern. Mayrhofer and Steinbereithner (15) have demonstrated major inaccuracies in the oxygen concentrations delivered by both *Bennett* and *Bird* ventilators, an observation of some considerable clinical implication. Mills (16) tested six different volume-regulated ventilators and was able to show significant residual volumes in test lungs under conditions of high airway resistance. He further found the alarm systems for both volume delivery and inspired oxygen concentration to be imperfect in all of them. International Standards Organization test procedures have been developed, designed to show up errors due to the internal compliance in the machine.

External influences of the most unusual and unsuspected nature can affect the performance of ventilators (8):

A 60-year-old male was being anaesthetized for cranioplasty. Anaesthesia was maintained with nitrous oxide, Innovar, and curare, and ventilation was controlled with a semi-closed circle absorber circuit by means of a 'Ventimeter' ventilator. The waste anaesthetic gases were being led to atmosphere by means of corrugated tubing from the exhalation valve of the ventilator to the air exhaust duct of the operating room. Part of this exhaust tubing was allowed to lie on the floor. During closure of the skull defect, the brain was observed to bulge and venous bleeding increased. At the same time the colour of the skin turned blue, and marked bradycardia was observed on the ECG monitor. A glance at the manometer on the soda-lime absorber showed that high pressures had developed in the circuit. It was then noted that one wheel of the anaesthetic machine had passed over the corrugated exhaust tubing. Relief of this obstruction was all that was needed for the operation to proceed to a successful conclusion (Fig. 36).

It is concluded that when this type of scavenging system is used and especially if compressible tubing is employed, a blow-off valve should be incorporated into the system proximal to any potential obstruction. Recognizing this same potential hazard, Bethune, Collis, and Latimer (6) have described a safety

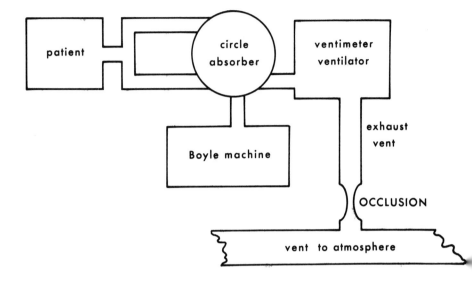

Figure 36 / Schematic drawing of occlusion of the scavenger exhaust vent leading to high pressure build-up.
From: Davies and Tarnawsky (8); *courtesy: Canadian Anaesthetists' Society Journal*

block which also provides a visual and auditory check on the functioning of the system.

Dunbar, Redick, and Merket (11) had the remarkable experience of encountering rapid inspiratory cycling regularly once every four hours for a period of five to seven seconds with an *Emerson Post Operative* ventilator. This coincided with the audio-frequency signal generated by a clock-setting system for the hospital. These audio-frequency bursts became superimposed on the AC current when clocks automatically reset themselves once every four hours. Similar interaction has been observed between the *Bourns Infant* ventilator (Model LS 105-150 and earlier models) and the Roche Model 1010 Arteriosonde (3), an arterial blood pressure measuring device. If the two instruments are placed in close proximity to each other, the magnet on the loudspeaker of the Arteriosonde can activate one or both magnetic reed switches which control the inspiratory and expiratory sequences and so prevent cycling. Merely increasing the distance between the two units beyond 15 cm will restore the ventilator to normal cycling.

HUMIDIFIERS AND NEBULIZERS

Very little can go wrong with the simple types of humidifiers, such as the *artificial nose*, and in any case malfunctions do not have serious consequences for the patient. Nor for that matter are they very efficient.

In more advanced models *thermostat failure* is a real problem as unduly hot water may cause burns of the respiratory tract. Overheating is an important hazard and several such incidents, some of them fatal, are known to have occurred (4). For that reason the incorporation of a second thermostat has been recommended. Ideally, what is needed is a cut-out controlled by a sensing thermostat at the airway.

Ultrasonic nebulizers, the latest addition to this type of equipment, are extremely efficient and must be controlled more closely than other apparatus in this category. There is a real danger of over-hydration of patients if the equipment is used indiscriminately. Such water intoxication can also occur with cold-mist humidifiers. El-Naggar, Collins, and Francis (5) point out that ultrasonic energy has great potential for localized heating and that a fire hazard exists in an oxygen enriched atmosphere. One such fire has occurred in their institution.

The *Aquatherm Aerosol heater unit* consists of the heater element with disposable water bottle and impact nebulizer. In the early model of this device leakage of water into the interior of the heater and electrical circuit portion of the equipment could occur, with consequent overheating of the element. When this happens, the unit stops operating and the intended aerosol is no longer delivered to the patient (1).

Conductors within the power cord of the *Ohio Immersion Heater* (Model DNH-1) have been known to break. This can cause arcing, smoke, melting, or even fire (2). A fire has also been reported when this same immersion heater was used in conjunction with the *Inspiron Disposable Nebulizer* (Model 002305) (3), because of the proximity of the heater barrel to the side of the plastic reservoir jar; tilting of the element caused by heat softening a plastic adaptor had caused this malalignment. A shock hazard exists with immersion heaters in case of ground wire breakage.

Finally condensation and accumulation of water in the inspiratory hose of a breathing circuit may impede gas flow.

RESUSCITATORS

Resuscitators can be divided roughly into those used in adults largely as part of emergency services and those used in the newborn. They are subject to the same kind of malfunctions as are ventilators, in the sense that lung ventilation may either be inadequate or over-inflation may occur.

When considering resuscitation equipment used in *adults*, one must remember that no one single resuscitator can suit all clinical conditions which call for resuscitation and be indicated in all environments, and that therefore different circumstances demand different performance characteristics. Another major consideration must be that this equipment is used to a large extent by unskilled or semi-skilled personnel, thus inviting a higher incidence of malfunctions and less expert assessment for exclusion of unsuitable or poorly performing equipment (1). Consequently such equipment should be mechanically as simple as possible. Based on this premise, Maggio and Vogelsanger (2) recommend that the EMO inhaler, in connection with the Oxford inflating bellows, is an efficient and safe apparatus. They do not recommend the use of the Ambu resuscitator particularly because the non-rebreathing valve may stick and the bag has no reservoir function. If however a bag with a reservoir capability is used, such as the Oxford inflating bellows, then a Ruben valve is acceptable. In some bags, such as the early AGA, flakes of rubber have been known to fall off the interior and jam the valves. They could even enter the respiratory tract.

In *neonatal resuscitation* the prime consideration must be that the pressures generated do not exceed accepted safe levels for lung expansion of the newborn. Williams, Beasley, and Fisher (4) in testing two resuscitators found that they did not conform to these basic requirements and, although changes have now been made by the manufacturers, it would seem appropriate for spot-checks to be made by those in charge of these apparati to make sure that they still conform to safety requirements even after they have been used for some time. Mathias (3) points out that care must be taken in the positioning of the water container so that water is not siphoned into the airway.

HYPOTHERMIA EQUIPMENT

Injury to patients because of malfunctioning equipment used for surface cooling is infrequent. Most are due to leaks of the cooling water from the blanket or one of its supply hoses. We have one such case on record:

Upon conclusion of the operation during which the temperature at the reservoir dropped to approximately −1 degree C, fluid was seen to drop off the foot end of the operating table. The source of the water was traced to a leak of one of the hoses leading to one of the blankets. When subsequently the patient was turned it was noted that her back was red and blistered, probably because she had been lying for some time in a pool of cold water. The second degree cold burns healed with conservative treatment. On testing the machine, no overt defect was detected and it was assumed that the leak in the hose was due to kinking and that the accompanying rise in pressure had forced water out of the joint.

Great care must be taken to prevent such accidents since serious scalds from either hot or cold water could result.

Obviously burns can result from the external application of excessive cold or for that matter heat. Probably the most common misadventure in this category are burns from hot water bottles applied to unconscious patients or to any part of the body rendered analgesic from whatever cause. However, burns can also result from the injudicious application of blankets containing perfusing coils which, while primarily intended for the induction and maintenance of hypothermia, may also be used as warming blankets. The following is a case in point:

A 65-year-old patient was undergoing sigmoid resection for diverticulitis. In the course of the operation the anaesthetist thought the patient felt somewhat cold. No action could be taken at that time. When the patient was returned to the Recovery Room he began to shiver and his oesophageal temperature was recorded at 34.5 degrees. Consequently application of a warming blanket was ordered. No detailed instructions were left with the nurses who placed the patient on a water-perfused blanket connected to a Therm-O-Rite hypo-hyperthermia unit. This is provided with a thermostat control graduated in an arbitrary scale of from 1 to 19, representing >51.3 degrees C (>150 degrees F) and -25 degrees C (12 degrees F) respectively. A chart converting the thermostat scale to actual temperatures is attached to each machine which also incorporates a thermometer indicating the temperature of the perfusing water. Without consulting the conversion chart the control was set at '1' in the erroneous belief that in doing so the least heating would be provided and no check of the water temperature was made. When the patient was later removed from the blanket it was found that he had suffered extensive third-degree burns on his back and calves which required repeated grafting procedures.

This is a case which was not due to any malfunction of the equipment but rather to the total ignorance of the personnel using it. Nevertheless, the manufacturer cannot be entirely exonerated for not having inscribed the thermostat dial directly with the temperature to be attained rather than with arbitrary numbers requiring reference to a separate explanatory label. The latest model of the equipment has an automatic thermally activated shut-off safety feature which causes the circulating pump to stop and a yellow light to flash whenever the heat transfer liquid exceeds 39 degrees C or falls below 2 degrees C. In further defence of the equipment it must be pointed out that mechanical stops are provided which are designed to prevent the pointers on the control thermostat knob from turning beyond certain predetermined positions. Unfortunately, the pointer may be broken off or the stops may have been unscrewed from the control panel, thus circumventing this particular safety measure. On the other hand, the absence of a backup thermostat in case of failure of the primary one is a definite safety hazard, one which other manufacturers of such equipment do provide (1, 2, 3, 4). Nevertheless, most complications arising out of the use of this equipment are due to human error, inattentiveness, or ignorance rather than equipment failure as such.

SPHYGMOMANOMETERS

Even such a relatively unsophisticated instrument as an ordinary sphygmomanometer can sometimes malfunction. It is, of course, well known that dropping of the aneroid meter may affect its zero setting, thus leading to erroneous readings. A bent needle may also affect the reading if it impinges upon the dial. Open mercury manometers may overflow under undue pressure, spilling mercury to the point where the reservoir may be depleted sufficiently to prevent the reading of high pressures.

A more disturbing complication is the sudden disappearance of any blood pressure readings whatsoever. This may be due to displacement of the stethoscope away from the site of the artery, but we havy one case on record in which this was due to twisting of the tubing of the stethoscope. The presence of a palpable pulse or heart sound will clarify the situation and avoid precipitate resuscitative actions.

PNEUMATIC TOURNIQUETS

Tourniquets which are inflated from a small compressed gas cylinder and of which the pressury can be regulated and maintained at a predetermined pressure have become standard equipment in recent years in many operating rooms for orthopaedic procedures and are used by anaesthetists for intravenous regional analgesia. One such instrument is shown in Figure 37A. The gas used to inflate the tourniquet could be carbon dioxide or, as in our case, dichlorodifluoromethane (FREON-12; 'Medic Air'). Again significant malfunctions other than the accidental deflation of the cuff can occur and the following is a case in point:

An intravenous regional block with a tourniquet in place was carried out for correction of a mallett finger. The operation had been in progress approximately

50 minutes when there was suddenly a loud explosive sound followed by hissing. Liquid 'Medic Air' was seen bubbling in the glass chamber which emptied rapidly accompanied by deflation of the tourniquet. A strong odour was perceived and was traced to the inflating gas. An ordinary tourniquet applied proximal to the site of the operation prevented the wearing off of the block. Inspection of the equipment showed that the rubber hose leading from the canister to the regulating valve had ruptured; hence the escape of the gas and tourniquet failure (Fig. 37B).

This particular instrument had been in service for a number of years and rubber fatigue was found to have been responsible for the failure. Some concern was expressed since the material is potentially toxic if inhaled in considerable concentration. Fortunately, the quantity of the gas used to inflate the tourniquet and the subsequent dilution in the ambient air nullified any danger to personnel.

It should also be remembered that the aneroid gauges of simpler pneumatic tourniquets are as vulnerable to damage as similar devices used for measuring blood pressure. Since they are dropped frequently, they should be tested regularly to avoid the obvious hazard of applying excess pressure.

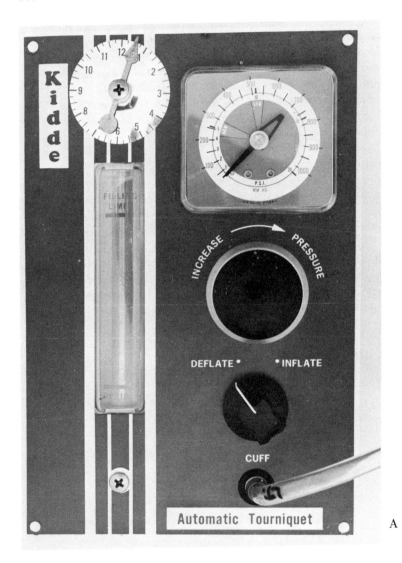

A

Figure 37 / A, Front panel of 'Kidde' automatic tourniquet.
B, Inside of 'Kidde' automatic tourniquet. Rupture of hose between cannister
and regulating valve led to tourniquet failure.

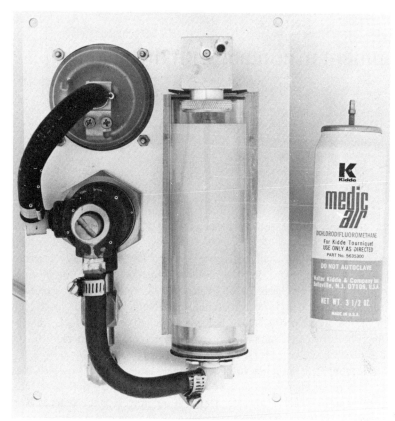

B

VI
Equipment in contact with the patient

AIRWAYS, MASKS, NASAL CATHETERS, AND MOUTHPIECES

Airways are not subject to malfunctions as long as they are properly inserted. However, care must be taken that the inside is properly cleaned, not so much because this is a basic requirement of hygiene or because there is a danger of obstruction, but rather that foreign material, including loose bits of plastic left over from the moulding process, may become detached and aspirated. Airways made from rubber or other semi-rigid material have a metal insert close to the outer flange to serve as a bite block. If lost, it must be replaced.

Masks also show little tendency to fail. The pneumatic cushion, however, may not retain air if the rubber is old and worn. Care must be taken that no residual chemical agents are retained from the sterilization process since this has been known to give rise to skin reactions or even burns at the site of contact.

The combustion of a *nasal catheter* carrying oxygen has been reported by Perel, Mahler, and Davidson (2). Ignition of the oxygen in this case was probably due to accumulation of static electrical charges made possible by a low relative humidity. While the bed was non-conductive, the nasal catheter through the humidified stream of oxygen served as conductor to the grounded oxygen outlet. The result would be a difference of potential between the insulated patient and the grounded catheter. The combustion of a tracheal tube while in use in the absence of flammable anaesthetics has also come to our attention.

Ball and Berry (1) have described a defect in the Juno Mark 2 disposable non-rebreathing *mouthpiece* used for self-administration of general analgesia, especially in obstetrical units. This mouthpiece contains a disc which serves as a one-way valve and is held in place by a retaining ring. As the mouthpiece warms from body contact, and especially after sterilization, a slight increase of its inner

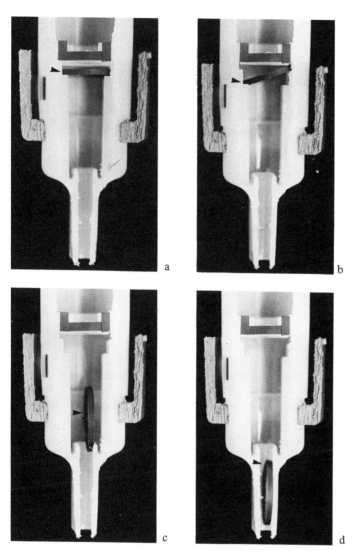

Figure 38 / Disposable non-rebreathing mouthpiece. a, Normal (arrow shows disc held in its normal position). b, Retaining shelf has moved allowing disc to tilt. c, Disc has fallen off retaining shelf, and d, has come to lie in the mouthpiece portion.

From: Ball and Berry (1); *courtesy: Anesthesiology*

diameter allows the ring to shift slightly and as a consequence the disc may dislodge and even slip into the patient's mouth (Fig. 38 a-d).

TRACHEAL TUBES

The tracheal tube is a flexible pipe which effects a direct connection between the trachea and the environment, anaesthetic machine, or ventilator, guarding the airway from obstruction by the soft tissues of the mouth and pharynx or from closure of the glottis. Tracheal tubes are most commonly made of red rubber, plastic, or latex reinforced with a helix of wire or nylon. They have a bevel at the patient end and just proximal to it they may be fitted with an inflatable cuff. Thus tracheal tubes are relatively simple devices without moving parts and one would not expect many misadventures because of mechanical failures. Yet such failures are frequent and indeed more common than with any other appliance used in anaesthesia. They were the cause of death in more than half the fatalities related to the breathing system in a study conducted in Australia (51). Although the tracheal tube is intended to provide free access of air to the lungs, paradoxically most misadventures arise because the same airway which it is intended to safeguard is being compromised because patency of the lumen is impaired. Obstructions may be intrinsic to the tracheal tube itself or extrinsic because of causes exerting their influence from outside. Other causes of failure may reside in the cuff mechanism without necessarily affecting patency of the tube. We shall, of course, not consider here malplacement of tracheal tubes which lead to their failure.

Since the tracheal tube is inserted for the specific purpose of maintaining a clear airway, an obstruction occurring from any cause can easily be overlooked unless the user is alert to this possibility. Like most anaesthetists we have on record numerous incidents of tracheal tube failures, including obstruction by mucus, blood clot, kinking, prolapsed cuffs, and impingement of the bevel against the tracheal wall.

Misadventures with tracheal tubes, however, are not limited to obstruction. Some old red rubber tubes have been found to become so brittle with age that they can easily be snapped into pieces. As a rule tubes should not be used if they are more than three years old, or at least they should be carefully examined for integrity before use, although shelf-life is somewhat influenced by storage conditions (18, 50). Phillips (75) describes an incident in which acute flexion of the tube showed a linear defect all along the attachment of the inflating tube from the cuff right to its machine end. It is recommended that every tube should be flexed prior to use to detect such defects. Chiu amd Meyers (21) found a punched-out area forming the Murphy eye of a sterile disposable polyvinyl chloride tube still in place. The punched-out piece yielded to pressure and fell into the lumen of the tube. Even a barb – a pin incorporated into its wall as a radiological marker – has been found protruding from the patient end of a tube (26). Since these defects in the manufacture were detected before use, no serious complications resulted, but these incidents again stress the need to inspect carefully every tracheal tube before insertion. Scheinfelder (85) lost a suction catheter down the tracheal tube during deep suction because of insecure connection to the vacuum line.

The tracheal tube itself can under some circumstances become a foreign body as described by Yeung and Lett (102) where, upon extubation, the entire distal latex portion of a four millimeter flexo-metallic tube was missing and had to be removed by bronchoscopy. MacIntosh (64) has made the point that deaths have occurred from entire tracheal tubes having been lost down the trachea in patients sent back to the ward with the tube in place, although usually this is not a fatal complication.

Finally some attention must be paid to the bevel of tracheal tubes, especially if they are to be used for nasal intubation, since it has been found that if the bevel is sharper than usual, the tube may find its way beneath the posterior pharyngeal mucosa (9, 24).

Intrinsic obstruction
Before a tube is inserted, its lumen must be examined for patency (8). Tracheal tubes have been found to be filled with blood and secretions (36, 40, 41, 43, 64). Clumps of debris and pus have been known to extend from the tube right on into a bronchus (5). In many of these instances obstruction was not complete and hence it was possible to pass a suction catheter through the tube while respiration was still markedly impaired.

Beyond this, a considerable variety of foreign bodies has been found in tracheal tubes from time to time (Fig. 39). Haselhuhn (46) found a rubber tip which normally covers the adaptor of an Abbott Venopack jammed tightly into the lumen. This, he assumed, was pushed down by the wire cleaning brush, while Jenkins (54) found part of a cleaning brush itself retained inside the lumen. Here again a stylet was passed and met with only slight resistance. Dutton (35) found a red rubber bung occluding the lumen, but since it had a small hole through which it allowed some air to pass, ventilation was possible albeit against considerable resistance. The presence of foam rubber hardened by inspissated sputum has been reported by Powell (77). The following case occurred in our hospital and is worth reporting in this connection:

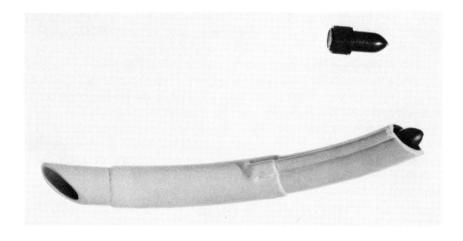

Figure 39 / Plug from inflating tube to mask cushion occluding tracheal tube lumen.
Courtesy: Dr K. Banton, University Hospital, Saskatoon

A 16-year-old girl was anaesthetized for pneumoencephalogram. Following tracheal intubation, there was some slight difficulty in inflating the lungs but this was not excessive and was thought to be due to light anaesthesia. Respirations were controlled for the first 45 minutes after which she was allowed to breathe spontaneously. Immediately it was noted then that there was 'vertical paradoxical' ('see-saw') respiration and the colour turned dusky for the first time. A suction catheter passed through the tube quite easily, yet the previous difficulty remained and on rechecking the tube some white material was seen within its lumen close to the machine end. Consequently the tube was replaced by another one. This immediately relieved all difficulties. On later inspection a piece of adhesive tape was found to occlude partially the lumen of the tracheal tube. In retrospect it was ascertained that a connector too small for that particular tube was used previously and in order to improve the fit, adhesive tape had been wound around its distal portion in an attempt to improve retention. When the connector was removed later and another one inserted the tape somehow had been left behind and had been pushed farther on by the second connector.

Peers (72) has referred to the presence of ampoule tops and needles inside the lumen of tracheal tubes in addition to blood clots and vomitus. He also describes a case in which the proximal rubber end of a Lenn's tube, a kind of gastric aspiration tube, was found within the lumen of a tracheal tube which had been used to guide the nasogastric tube into the stomach on a previous occasion. In another case (4) the cuff was torn and approximately half of it had invaginated itself into the lumen of the tracheal tube, thus acting as a ball-valve.

Even tubes which have been pre-checked and found patent may become obstructed during use. The following incident from our files illustrates this well:

A 10-month-old infant was anaesthetized for correction of esotropia in the left eye. Tracheal intubation was carried out with a 3-mm Cole tracheal tube and was quite uneventful. Shortly after the start of the operation some harsh rasping noises began to appear in the airway, but since the face was tightly draped and no indrawing was noted, this was considered not of sufficient importance to disturb the surgeon and risk possible contamination of the operative field. The anaesthetic proceeded uneventfully for the next 20 minutes, but then complete respiratory obstruction suddenly occurred and could not be relieved by manipulation of the tube under the drapes. Consequently, the tube was removed and anaesthesia maintained by applying the mask as close to the face of the infant as possible without interfering with the surgical field. Later, inspection of the tube showed that the distal one cm was completely obstructed by inspissated secretions (Fig. 40) which must have accumulated rapidly in the course of some 20 minutes, the time that had elapsed from the first occurrence of sound in the airway, to the point of total obstruction. There had been no clinical signs of any respiratory infection in this infant other than a small crust at the right nostril which was noted before induction of anaesthesia but was considered insignificant in view of the absence of clinical signs.

Pelagio and associates (73) report airway obstruction during pneumonectomy due to a friable mass which had entered both the tracheal tube and the main stem bronchus. Tofany (96) relates the case of a twenty-two months old baby whose tracheal tube became obstructed during thoracotomy for removal of a bronchial foreign body and was found plugged by granulation tissue likely forced into the end of the tube during expiration.

Tracheal intubation by the nasal route is another way in which a previously patent tube may become obstructed. In children adenoid tissue may be picked up. For that reason nasal intubation is avoided in children if at all possible. In one case reported in the literature (3) tissue was severed from the nasal choana by the tube, entered its lumen and so became the cause of obstruction in addition to inflicting severe trauma.

Finally, a rather unique case of obstruction of a tracheal tube has been described by Mimpriss (67) who found an ascaris doubled back on itself and acting as a non-return valve causing extensive surgical emphysema. He warns

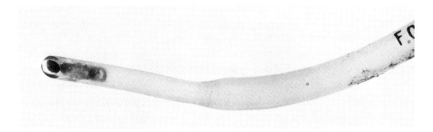

Figure 40 / Tracheal end of Cole tracheal tube completely occluded by inspissated secretions.

against this occurrence in areas in which ascaris is endemic, and where the parasite has been known not infrequently to find its way into the airway.

Reinforced tracheal tubes have inherent dangers of intrinsic obstruction of their own because of the method of their manufacture. These tubes consist of a helical matrix which is covered by latex. This is applied through a process of repeated dipping. Drying takes place after each dipping. Because of this it is possible for layering to occur and consequently complete or partial separation of these layers is a possibility.

Separation of the inner layer may result in blister formation where an air-space exists between two separate layers of latex. With exposure to anaesthetics the inner layer may swell leading to obstruction (16), but blister formation has also been reported after ethylene oxide sterilization (14). The blisters may disappear in time, but light patches indicate the existence of two separate layers with airspace between them. In a case described by Kohli and Manku (60) an interesting situation arose when air from the cuff managed to escape between two layers and into the bevel of a reinforced tube. During expiration, air from the cuff had free access to the defect between the layers, while positive pressure on inspiration pushed the air back into the cuff. Hence, partial obstruction and wheezing were heard only during expiration, mimicking bronchospasm. A similar case has been described by Bachand and Fortin (6) in which a bulge developed at the bevelled extremity of the tube where the metal spirals do not extend. The air from the inflated cuff infiltrated between the two layers of latex, thus creating an unsupported inflated extension of the cuff, with the result that airway obstruction occurred. When the air was released from the cuff, the deflation of the ballooned extension flap was slow. A case has been described by Ng and Kirimli (70) in which intralumenal herniation occurred from the intramural cuff inflating tube of a reinforced tracheal tube at the site where the 15-mm connector impinges against the cuff inflating tube at its entry into the tube wall, while an aneurysmal dilatation of the inflating tube into the lumen of the tracheal tube caused total obstruction whenever the cuff was inflated in a case cited by Abramowitz and McNabb (1).

Walton (97) describes two tubes which contained rubbery material, likely residuals from manufacture, which caused almost complete obstruction. Moreover, pieces might come loose and be aspirated. Another author has reported the distal part of a reinforced latex tube to have become invaginated with consequent reduction of the lumen (98). This might have occurred when the cleaning brush was withdrawn. In another experience, Blitt (12) found thin filmy membranes at several levels of the lumen. Since reinforced tubes must be introduced with the help of a stylet, which in his case had been lubricated with two per cent lidocaine jelly, it is believed that some of this material adhered to the wall of the tube and then dried with the passage of dry gases. This formed a film. The use of a teflon stylet without lubrication is recommended. Other such stylets which do not require lubrication have been described by Linder (63) and Marshall (66).

Extrinsic obstruction
All anaesthetists would agree that one of the very common causes of obstruction of tracheal tubes is kinking. This usually occurs at points where the tube undergoes marked changes in direction and especially so if the head is acutely flexed or just distal to the patient end of the adaptor, especially if the tube is too tightly stretched over it (7, 8, 61). While this event is most common with rubber or plastic tubes, it has been known to occur also with reinforced tubes. They can kink at the machine end if the connector is not advanced into the reinforced portion of the tube (7, 61). In order to overcome this disadvantage, Hale Enderby recommends the use of a tapered tube in which the reinforced portion can be brought up all the way to the machine end of the tube and yet permit insertion of a connector of such size as not to reduce the lumen to any significant degree (44, 45).

Nasotracheal tubes made of rubber commonly have a lesser wall thickness than tubes for oral use in order to provide the largest possible internal diameter. Since the thinner wall renders the tube more liable to kinking, a danger much reduced if the nasal route is used, it follows that such tubes are unsuitable for oral intubation. We know of at least one death because this restriction was ignored.

Tubes may also become obstructed because of teeth biting on the rubber if a bite block has not been inserted (7). Adamson (2) has described a case in which the patient even bit through a reinforced tube with his incisors and canines, compressing it at the same time with his molars in yet another area. At the patient end the soft tip of a reinforced tube may become bent and thus obstruct. Our department has one case on record in which the adhesive tape used to hold the tube in place exerted undue tension on the tracheal tube causing it to be flattened. The result was partial airway obstruction.

Careful attention must be paid to the integrity of the tube since repeated boiling and autoclaving softens the walls of tubes, thus making them more subject to kinking (93). Bosomworth and Hamelberg (14) have shown that, in general, red rubber tubes kink more readily than clear plastic ones and this difference is retained after repeated boiling and steam sterilization. On the other hand, plastic tubes are more readily compressed than rubber ones. They found that boiling and steam sterilization are the most hazardous in this regard, with ethylene oxide being intermediate, while hexachlorophene and benzylkonium chloride are the least harmful both for tubes and cuffs.

External pressure has also been known to affect plastic tubes at the site of the tracheal cuff if this is inflated. Price (78) found some new tubes to be thinner in the area underlying the cuff. A rise in temperature from 15 to 37° C causes an increase of pressure within the cuff of approximately 10 per cent which, in turn, can lead to partial compression of the lumen. Furthermore, increased temperature raises the compliance of polyvinyl chloride tubes (57). Sobel (89), after removing a leaking cuff from a plastic tracheal tube, observed that underneath the region of the cuff there was an area of constriction 2¼ inches long where the thermolabile plastic apparently had become remodelled by body warmth and that the upper 3/4 inch of this area was indeed buckled in. Rollason (83) also has stressed that the initial inflating pressure in cuffs should be only moderate and just adequate for an air-tight fit since pressure of the air in the cuff rises as it reaches body temperature in accordance with the coefficient of expansion. Stanley (90, 91, 86) has demonstrated that nitrous oxide diffuses into the cuff and so increases the volume of a latex cuff by 30 to 40 per cent in one hour and 60 per cent nitrous oxide diffuses also into polyvinylchloride cuffs. The increased pressure may cause collapse of the tube, especially in view of the fact that marked variances in firmness have been found in different lots (57). Wong (100) has experienced the actual collapse of a disposable polyvinyl chloride tracheal tube under the cuff (Fig. 41) and so have Roland and Stovner (82). They were able to reproduce the collapse shortly after extubation by inflating the cuff with 8 ml of air. Generally they have shown that at 37 degrees C polyvinyl tubes tend to collapse with cuff pressures between 310 and 460 mmHg (41.2-61.2 kPa). With the diffusion of nitrous oxide and carbon dioxide at 3.69 volumes per cent and 0.36 volume per cent per hour respectively, increases of the cuff pressure to such dangerous levels can be produced in the

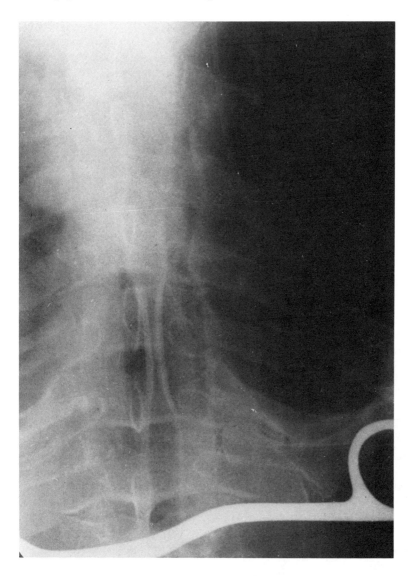

Figure 41 / Collapse of tracheal tube under cuff.
From: Dr R.M. Wong (100); *courtesy: Anaesthesia and Intensive Care*

course of a long operation. They recommend that cuffs should be deflated periodically during anaesthesia to avoid this complication. This can also be achieved by following the lead of Stanley, Foote, and Liu (92) who have devised a valve which prevents increase in volume of and pressure within the cuff while maintaining an airtight seal. Alternatively the cuff might be inflated with a sample of the inspired anaesthetic mixture (6, 100). That overinflation of high-compliance cuffs also can compromise the lumen of tracheal tubes has been reported by Perel and associates (74). Hoffman and Freeman have summed up the causes of tracheal tube collapse as a combination of many factors, namely frequent use, softening of the tube wall by body heat, gradual increase of intra-cuff volume, and pressure by diffusion of nitrous oxide into the cuff, replacement of a damaged cuff by a new one, and heat sterilization (49).

Even reinforced tracheal tubes can become obstructed by pressure from without. Nylon does not have a high resistance to compression and in consequence two cases of respiratory obstruction have occurred when the laryngoscope blade compressed nylon-reinforced tracheal tubes during microlaryngoscopy (20). It is anticipated that recent modifications in the manufacturing process will prevent such occurrences in the future (76). Alternatively the cuff may be the offending agent, as when softening and distortion of the nylon spirals result if the cuff is inflated during sterilization by boiling (53). Others have found this to be due to weakness in the inner surface of the latex which can give way (38, 80). Catane and Davidson (19) have reported that inflation of the cuff when external pressure was applied to it could lead to ballooning of the inner layer of the tube with the result that complete obstruction of the lumen occurred.

Clark (23) has warned of the danger of obstruction of tracheal tubes due to over-inflation of the cuff. Cohen and Dillon (25) have described four cases of obstruction. Uneven dilatation of the cuff causes eccentric displacement of the tube. If the dilatation is on the side away from the bevel, it will cause the bevel to impinge against the wall of the trachea. If expansion is on the side towards which the bevel faces, the tip of the bevel itself may become occluded by the bulging cuff (Fig. 42). Examples of the former have been described by Mirakhur (68) and by Pryer, Pryer, and Williams (79), while many examples of herniation over the end of the tube also are known (31, 99) and many more have been experienced in everyday practice. In many instances this is due to over-inflation of a weakened cuff.

Laryngeal microsurgery was being done under tracheal intubation around a small-born cuffed tracheal tube. During placement of the laryngoscope the tube was slightly withdrawn and this resulted in complete obstruction. A defect was later detected in that the distal insertion of the cuff at one point reached the

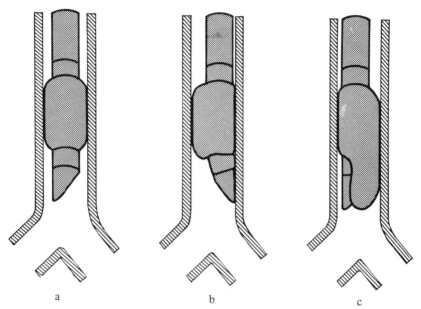

Figure 42 / a, Normal position of tracheal tube within the trachea; even inflation of cuff. b, Eccentric inflation of the cuff forcing the bevel against the tracheal wall. c, Eccentric inflation of the cuff on the side of the bevel leading to occlusion of the bevel.

level of the bevel, an error that was responsible for this mishap (42). Also the lower end of a tracheal tube can be drawn into the cuff (10) if the tube is pulled back while the cuff is inflated and is being firmly held against the wall of the trachea. This is especially likely to happen if the portion of the tube projecting beyond the cuff is short. The dimensions specified in the ISO draft standard of tracheal tubes are intended to prevent or at least minimize this hazard.

In the case described by Hedden, Smith, and Torpay (48) the obstruction was caused by the end of the tube being forced against the wall of the trachea. This was aggravated by severe scoliosis while the patient had a Risser jacket applied under general anaesthesia in the prone position. Liew (62) explains the obstruction of an Oxford tube when the head and neck are flexed acutely, as in the sitting position for neurosurgical procedures, by the posteriorly directed bevel impinging against the posterior tracheal wall. Salt (84) recommends that a hole equal in size to the cross section of the tube be cut in its anterior wall when occlusion of the airway from this cause is anticipated. If a double-walled slip-on cuff is incorrectly applied to the tracheal tube so that the inner wall is allowed to slip beneath the constricting band of the cuff, inflation with volumes of air intended to give a gas-tight fit will cause the inner wall to herniate, forcing the bevel of the tube against the trachea. This particular situation is not remedied by allowing air to escape from the cuff since its shoulder acts as a one-way valve and prevents the herniation from emptying (87). Rollason (83) has made the point that leaks or herniation are best detected if the cuff is inflated inside a test tube.

Another cause of obstruction could be the impinging of the tip of the tube on the carina and its being folded over into the lumen of the tube (25).

Tracheal cuffs

Apart from their effect on the patency of the tube, mechanical failure of cuffs themselves has been known to occur. Bursting of the cuff during use is particularly disconcerting when, on removal, it is found that a piece of the cuff is missing. Sometimes this can be removed by suction from the trachea but at other times bronchoscopy may be required (27, 30, 32, 58, 88). It is often not realized that rubber deteriorates when grease or oil is applied to it and such treatment, as well as frequent sterilization, may predispose to distortion or bursting. Consequently, it is recommended that only water-base lubricants be used on tracheal tubes and cuffs (15).

Another complication in the use of tracheal cuffs relates to inability to deflate them before extubation. This has been seen not infrequently in cuffed reinforced tubes with embedded inflating tubes. It is peculiar to this type of tracheal tube and cannot be duplicated in a Magill tube, in that the inflation tube is caught between the first spiral and the tracheal tube connector, thus preventing the escape of air from the cuff (86). As previously pointed out, the connector must be advanced to the first spiral to prevent kinking of the soft machine end of the tube. The same mechanism of compression of the inflating tube can also prevent inflation of the cuff and should be suspected if the pilot balloon expands unduly, yet a seal of the cuff to the tracheal wall cannot be effected (11, 65). However, Dunn (34) has pointed out that slight traction upon the connector permits inflation, while deflation still cannot be guaranteed.

If forceps are used to occlude inflating tubes made of latex, the tube walls often stick together, thus preventing deflation of the cuff. Another mechanism of obstruction of the inflation tubes has been described by Gould and Seldon (43) in an ordinary non-reinforced tube. It is believed that the bulging balloon had pressed the tracheal tube against the wall of the trachea, thus squeezing the inflating tube and closing it off. Carrie (17) has drawn attention to the fact that in some tubes two small slits are cut into the inflating tube as it passes through

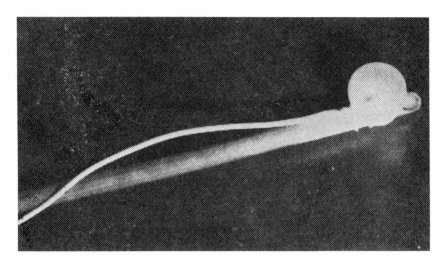

Figure 43 / Tracheal tube with bolus of air trapped in the distal portion
of the cuff.
Courtesy: New York State Medical Journal 56: 3937 (1956)

the pilot balloon. These slits can become occluded in certain positions so that
the pilot balloon does not inflate with the cuff. This might be interpreted as
non-inflation of the cuff with consequent potential overinflation on a second
injection of air. Alternatively, if the slits close later the cuff might become
deflated while the pilot balloon remains distended.

A rather interesting case has been described by Davies (28) affecting a reinforced latex tracheal tube. In construction of such a tube it is dipped in latex
once more after the cuff has been applied to bind it to the tube. This last layer
may not fuse with the cuff and when inflation is made, air may pass around the
inflated cuff through a small defect and become trapped between the two layers.
When the cuff is deflated, the real inner cuff deflates but the outer shell remains
distended with air trapped in it. Another case of non-deflation of the cuff has
been reported by Koch and Franke (59). Here complete deflation of the cuff
was prevented because it had come to lie within the larynx. Traumatic laryngitis
strangulated the inflated cuff. On deflation, the part of the cuff below the glottis
remained inflated and had to be punctured with a lumbar-puncture needle before
extubation could be completed. In yet another instance (3) a bolus of air was
trapped in the distal portion of the cuff and was so placed that it could not
escape when the inflating tube was opened. It also partially occluded the end of
the tube and probably the left main bronchus (Fig. 43).

Blott (13) has described an instance of complete respiratory obstruction during pneumonectomy in which it was found that the slip-on cuff had become detached from the tube. It is likely that during suction the tube was withdrawn one-half to one inch, leaving the cuff behind with its inner wall closing over the end of the tube.

Elliott (37) has encountered two cases. In one of them deflation of the cuff was impeded because the patient had bitten on the inflating tube causing it to become sealed. The second tube had a cuff filled with polyurethane foam. Unlike ordinary cuffs these are permanently distended and are deflated by the evacuation of air. In this particular case the distal part of the inflating tube had become avulsed so that the cuff refilled spontaneously, and remained so since no means of air aspiration remained. Tavacoli and Corssen (95) had a similar experience with a self-inflatable 'Bivona' tracheal tube cuff, but Kamen and Wilkinson point out that this tube may be removed without deflation since the cuff will collapse as it is gently pulled out past the vocal cords (56). It is claimed that doing so may indeed be of benefit since secretions above the cuff are thus effectively removed. 'Flange' formation in the form of a collar-like ridge at the distal end of standard cuffs may be another cause of difficulty with extubation (69). Flange formation is more likely to occur in old or worn tubes.

Wong has encountered a rather rare defect in which deflation of the cuff occurred after a satisfactory seal with the trachea had existed for one and a half hours (101). Examination of the Portex Blueline polyvinyl chloride tube revealed air-bubbles issuing from its distal extremity when it was immersed in water (Fig. 44). The source of this leak was traced to a small hole in the end of the inflating channel which is moulded into the wall of this tube and extends beyond the cuff.

In other instances cuffs have failed to distend adequately or not at all thus preventing an air-tight seal. Debnath and Waters (29) describe two cases of separation of the attached margins of cuffs so that aspiration would have been possible, while Tahir and Adriani (94) describe two other cases in which large quantities of air failed to effect a seal by causing deformity of the contour of the trachea. This seems to be a property of cuffs made of low compliance rubber. However, Pavlin, Van Nimwegan, and Hornbein (71) have described a case in which a high compliance low-pressure cuff also failed to prevent aspiration.

Doubled-lumen tubes

These tubes are subject to many of the same difficulties which have been described for ordinary tracheal tubes. For instance, Clarke (22) found that the lumen of such a tube could become obstructed by inward pressure of the tracheal cuff. One case described by Jenkins (55) is more specific for double-

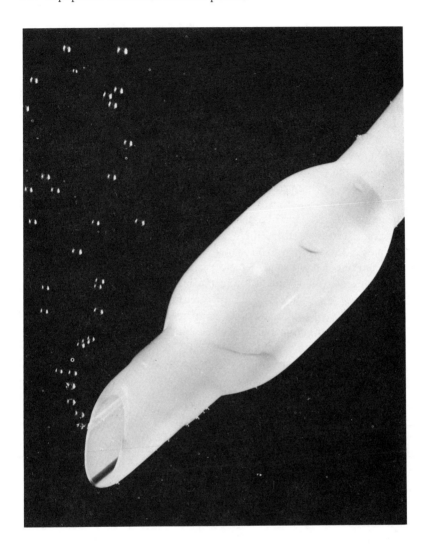

Figure 44 / Air bubbles from distal end of open inflating tube.
From: Dr R.M. Wong (101); *courtesy: Anaesthesia and Intensive Care*

lumen cuffs. The inflating tubes were wrongly labelled so that the tracheal cuff inflated when inflation of the bronchial cuff was intended and vice versa. Hayes (47) has described a structural defect in the wall of some Carlens tubes which can be felt by palpation through the proximal cuff. Even moderate distention with air produces collapse of the tube on one side, leading to partial or complete obstruction of the airway on the affected side. Hudson and Ross (52) have described an unusual defect in a Robertshaw tube in which a narrow slit existing in the septum between the two lumena caused a persistent leak when only one lung was being ventilated. So far all misadventures due to human error have been those caused by the anaesthetist. That the surgeon, working in the immediate vicinity of anaesthetic equipment may also unwittingly cause equipment to fail is illustrated by a case reported by Dryden (33). Here in the course of a left pneumonectomy, the surgeon had placed a suture through the anterior wall of the Carlens tube just above the spur. When the tube was removed, albeit somewhat vigorously, the suture was broken freeing the pulmonary artery. Shock supervened and the patient died. In another case, a bronchial cuff herniated across the carina distending and splitting the bronchial stump (103). Franklin (39, 81) has drawn attention to significant variations in the length of the bronchial segments in some Robertshaw tubes compared to earlier models. While this is not a malfunction of equipment as such, it could have significant impact on anaesthetic management in a particular patient and points to the necessity of developing standards for as many items of equipment as possible even in the face of major difficulties in their formulation.

TRACHEOSTOMY TUBES

Tracheostomy tubes are subject to many of the hazards which have been described for tracheal tubes other than those, of course, which relate to their position within the oral cavity.

Foreign bodies other than dried mucus are rare in tracheostomy tubes and are even less likely now with the more common use of disposable tubes. But even if the tube has been checked for patency, a foreign body may still become lodged within it as described by Röse (8). His patient was unconscious from a head injury and had a tracheostomy done on the second day. Soon after the tube had been inserted there was a bout of coughing followed by total respiratory obstruction. The tube was changed and it was found that it had become blocked by a broken tooth which must have been aspirated at the time of the injury and was thrown into the tube by the coughing spell.

As with tracheal tubes, complications from defective cuffs are not uncommon. These are most often due to herniation of the cuff (5, 6, 9) and not infrequently are associated with improper pre-stretching. Not only do such herniated cuffs displace the tracheostomy tube, but they have been known to bulge over the tracheal opening, obstructing it partially or completely. In this connection it should be remembered that tracheostomy tubes, unlike tracheal tubes, do not have bevelled patient ends. Only tracheostomy tubes with built-in cuffs should be used. Slip-on cuffs, especially when applied to metal tubes, are quite dangerous since they have been known to slip off the tube and, if inflated, may cause total respiratory obstruction.

Berkebile and Smith (1) describe a case in which the patient was unable to breathe around the occluded tracheostomy tube after the cuff had been deflated and the pilot balloon was down. The situation was remedied after the residual air had been aspirated from the pre-stretched cuff. Such cuffs are prone to deflate incompletely unless air is actively removed.

Similar difficulties have been experienced when attempts were made to withdraw some types of 'Portex' tracheostomy tubes (7). In some instances this has even necessitated enlargement of the stoma before extubation could be accomplished. The plastic balloon cuff in these cases had failed to collapse completely when deflated because it had become stiffened by the absorption of moisture. Incubation of these tubes in water at body temperature has shown that cuffs turn white within 24 hours with rigid circular structures forming at the distal and proximal ends of the cuffs. These 'flanges' offer considerable resistance and are the reasons for the difficulty experienced in extubation. Within 30 minutes of concluding the experiment the changes in the cuff had receded. This defect in cuff performance which has been demonstrated in older tubes with somewhat thicker cuffs than are now being produced is being remedied in more recent versions of 'Portex' tubes.

Relative newcomers to the equipment scene are plastic swivel connectors, both of the autoclavable and of the disposable type. They have been examined for leaks by Holdcroft, Loh, and Lumley (3) who found a leak exceeding 5 per cent of gas flow in the autoclavable type. The disposable and older metal varieties, however, were found to be acceptable. Leaks were found to vary with the position of the connector on the tube adaptor and were diminished after autoclaving. Unfortunately, this also reduced greatly the ease of swivelling. In a later study (4), leaks from Portex models had been reduced to the more acceptable level of less than 2 per cent with continuous and intermittent gas flows of 9 l/min., but another manufacturer's product was still unacceptable.

Ware (10) has drawn attention to a difficulty that arises when a Portex soft-seal tracheostomy tube is used with a swivel connector. He has found that in several instances the sealing ring on the tube has become detached when lateral force was used to separate the two components and the ring was retained inside the connector. When this occurs re-connection is impossible and both tracheostomy tube and connector must be changed. While changes are being made by the manufacturers to obviate such occurrences, many of the older assemblies will be part of hospital stocks for a considerable time even after the improved models become commercially available.

Finally Chamney (2) has pointed out that heat and moisture exchangers may become obstructed if the patient coughs up lumps of mucus, as indeed may also happen to the tube itself.

LARYNGOSCOPES

Failures of laryngoscopes relate largely to the light source. Most laryngoscopes used by anaesthetists are battery-operated and it is therefore essential that they be checked before operation to ensure that the light works and is of adequate intensity.

While bulbs may burn out, a more common cause of total light failure is a loose connection which simply requires that the bulb be screwed more firmly into its seat. Many laryngoscope blades are of the hook-on type and poor contact between handle and blade may be another source of light failure. In old blades the thread of the bulb seat may be worn, thus leading to precarious contact. Adequate light may be present when the instrument is tested, but the bulb may be moved by contact with the patient's tongue and so light may be lost. Such instruments obviously must be repaired or discarded.

No reference has been found in the literature of light bulbs becoming totally detached from the laryngoscope and being lost into the patient, although theoretically this could occur.

MAGILL FORCEPS AND LARYNGEAL SPRAYS

Only one case of breakage of a Magill forceps has been described in the literature (1). In that particular case tracheal intubation was carried out by the nasal route under direct vision. When later the surgeon exposed the lesion in the mouth, a semi-circular fragment some five millimeters long and two to three millimeters wide was seen at the base of the tongue and retrieved. This piece of metal was identified as part of the Magill forceps. Fortunately it was seen and removed while the tube was still in place so that aspiration was prevented.

Difficulties with laryngeal sprays have been described more frequently. A most serious potential hazard of early types was that they could syphen streams of liquid anaesthetic into the throat. Two fatalities from this cause occurred in 1939 (2).

Francis (4) described a case where the nozzle of the spray had become detached at laryngoscopy and had passed unnoticed into the pharynx and oesophagus. It was subsequently removed at laparotomy from the large bowel where its progress had become arrested. Paymaster (6) describes a serious potential hazard of the MacIntosh laryngeal spray in which the plastic tip can become detached from the inner tubing to which in his particular model it was fixed by means of a thread only. While the tip was not lost in this case, nevertheless the danger exists that this might occur. Lastly Liew (5) has drawn attention to the ease with which the nozzle of an Astra spray bottle can become detached if the hole in the plastic mount into which it is plugged has become worn through use. In one of his cases this indeed did occur and the nozzle disappeared between the cords, but luckily could be removed by suction. Evers (3), in commenting on this hazard, has remarked that loss of retention may be due to the fact that nozzles have not been allowed to cool after heat sterilization. As the hot nozzle is inserted, melting of the valve part of the bottle is a possibility. This in turn would enlarge the retaining hole. Disposable plastic nozzles have been made available to obviate this hazard.

NEEDLES FOR INJECTION

Needles may become blocked, bent, or broken. The most common site for breakage is where the shaft of the needle joins the hub. For that reason needles should never be inserted so far that only the hub protrudes from the skin since, should the needle break, it will disappear below the skin and this may make surgical removal necessary. Such a procedure could be complex if the needle were to travel within the vein or if the accident should occur with a spinal puncture needle. Insertion close to joints is equally hazardous as the following case illustrates:

A general anaesthetic was induced for forceps extraction in the delivery room. Before induction with gaseous agents, a needle was inserted into a vein in the antecubital fossa and a Gordh mount was attached to it. Induction was somewhat stormy and in the course of it the patient moved her arms. When later the anaesthetist attempted to inject an oxytocic, the Gordh mount had disappeared and was eventually found lying on the floor with the hub of the needle still attached (Fig. 45). Luckily, in this case the needle could be felt subcutaneously and after application of a tourniquet was easily removed.

The point has been made by many authors that, at least for regional anaesthesia, only security needles which incorporate a bead distal to the junction of the

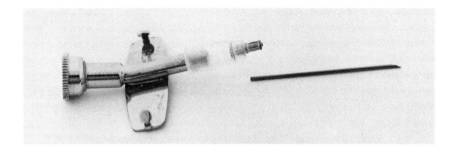

Figure 45 / Gordh needle mount with needle broken off at the hub.

needle to the hub should be used (2, 3, 9, 10, 12). The introduction of disposable needles has introduced a new hazard, namely that the plastic hub may become detached from the metal shaft (6, 11).

In 1966 Charlebois drew attention to *coring* as a major hazard in anaesthesia, as indeed it is in all facets of medicine (4). He showed in a series of tests carried out with 16 and 17 gauge needles that coring occurs whenever a hollow needle perforates any surface, whether this be skin or a diaphragm. A piece of the material roughly the size of the inside diameter of the needle is punched out and may then be injected into the patient. Coring of skin is of great significance when injection is to be made into the epidural or subarachnoid space and therefore it is advisable to use a stylet or first to make a hole in the skin with a needle larger than the one used for the actual puncture. The Sise introducer is useful for this purpose. By the same token, coring may occur by piercing a diaphragm. This is the case when drugs are aspirated from multi-dose vials.

Although Charlebois was the first to study the problem systematically, it had not escaped the attention of earlier investigators. Magath and McLellan (8) experimented with neoprene and synthetic rubber plugs in guinea-pigs. They found that when injected into tissues they produced only relatively mild foreign body reactions, but that consequences were more serious if they were injected into a blood vessel or became a nidus for infection. In order to avoid coring, they recommend that needles with lateral openings are preferable to end-open ones. This recommendation has been supported by Gibson and Morris (7), but they suggest that trocar-pointed side-open needles as described by Crawford Little (5) need only be used when it is desirable, for any reason, to avoid the risk of skin emboli. After all, experience with end-open needles in many millions of cases over many years has obviously shown that in the majority of cases the risk of complications from coring is negligible, although its incidence has been shown to be 69 per cent. More recently Baillie and Catton (1) have drawn attention to the fact that coring may also occur when the introducer of an intravenous infusion set pierces the diaphragm which occludes the solution-carrying container. The core observed in the solution by these authors could easily have passed through a number of 16 Argyle Medicut and thence into the patient's circulation.

INTRAVENOUS CANNULAE AND CATHETERS

Intravenous cannulae have become increasingly popular in recent years and have to a large degree replaced needles for the establishment of intravenous infusions. While most current cannulae are made of plastic or nylon rather than metal and are inserted outside the introducing needle, long intravenous catheters must be inserted through the lumen of a needle larger in diameter than that of the catheter. Consequently, there is a danger that the catheter may be sheared off by the sharp bevel of the needle if, in order to overcome any obstacle to its advance, it is manipulated in any direction other than forward (13). We have one case on record in which a central venous pressure catheter was sheared off on partial withdrawal while the inducing needle was still in place:

A central venous pressure catheter was inserted via the right antecubital fossa in preparation for resection of coarction of the aorta. Since the drip had slowed down as the catheter was being advanced, it was withdrawn slightly and it became obvious immediately that it had been sheared off at the bevel. A cut-down was done over the basilic vein well above the site where the x-ray had revealed the end of the catheter. Despite the fact that a tourniquet had been applied, the end of the catheter was only just visible in the operative area by the time it had been reached.

Cannulae which are introduced over the needle are, of course, not subject to the same danger. However, some materials become brittle and therefore have been known to break. In either case catheter emboli may form and be transported away from the site of insertion towards the right heart and beyond. Short catheters are used for the establishment and maintenance of intravenous infusions while long ones are employed for central venous pressure measurements, femoral, cardiac, or pulmonary artery catheterization.

Catheters may break for a number of reasons other than those mentioned. Al-Abrak and Samuel (1) cite an instance in which a central venous pressure catheter broke at the site of puncture when an attempt was made to remove it. X-rays showed that the catheter had looped within the vein and by pulling on it had tightened the loop causing fixation and eventual breakage. In another case described by Coppel and Samuel (7) the catheter had passed up the cephalic vein into the subclavian and then had backed into the arm via the axillary. The acute bend had made it difficult to remove the stilette and on one attempt the catheter itself had become frayed. Kinking is, indeed, one of the more common causes of breakage (14). Should a catheter break and the break occur in an extremity, the application of a tourniquet proximal to the foreign body should be applied to prevent its onward migration (28).

In the prevention of external breakage of catheters it has been recommended that they be secured properly, especially those introduced through a needle when the needle is left in situ. The tip of the needle should be covered by a guard (16). Where an open cut-down is done, the catheter should be securely tied to the vein and sutured to the skin (30).

Should catheter embolization occur (8, 32), removal is almost always indicated because of the danger of associated thrombi, the possibility of bacterial endocarditis, bacteraemia, or thrombophlebitis, to prevent recurrent pericardial effusions, to decrease the incidence of myocardial or coronary vessel damage, and because of psychoneurosis (11, 19, 29). On the whole, infection of lost catheters is more harmful than the embolus itself, and they should be removed in all cases. Many methods of removal have been described, from open cardiotomy (3, 10), transvenous removal from the right atrium by means of an alligator-jawed endoscopic forceps inserted through the right external jugular vein (24), to the use of a snare advanced through the venous system. This latter method is the one presently preferred (12, 18, 20, 21).

The danger of not searching for a lost catheter is well illustrated by Brown and Kent (4). In this case a catheter lost during prolonged intravenous therapy migrated from the femoral vein and perforated the right ventricle more than two months later, leading to cardiac tamponade and death.

Apart from breakage, knotting of catheters has been reported by a number of authors (15, 25). It has been pointed out that if a knot occurs in a flow-directed balloon catheter and fluoroscopy is not available, ventricular dysrhythmias are highly suggestive that knotting has occurred. In most instances it should be possible to withdraw the knotted catheter and replace it without much difficulty. Swaroop (26) has described an interesting situation in which a central venous pressure catheter was passed, followed later by a pulmonary artery catheter to measure both pressures in an effort to regulate fluid balance. Pulmonary artery pressure recordings were discontinued 24 hours later and on withdrawing the pulmonary artery catheter it was found to be tied in a knot with the central venous pressure catheter. The knot could not be undone under fluoroscopy. It was pulled into the right axillary vein to be removed by cutdown under local analgesia. Not even a stylet within a catheter guarantees that knotting will not occur. One such 32.4 cm long 'inside needle' central venous catheter was inserted into the superior vena cava via the internal jugular vein. When in position just proximal to the right atrium an attempt was made to withdraw the stylet, but without success. Thereupon the entire catheter was removed, but when its tip had reached the subcutaneous tissue, further withdrawal was impossible until a small skin incision had been made. Examination revealed a tight knot in the distal part of the catheter with the stylet still in situ (9).

Recently Talmage (27) has described yet another hazard of intra-arterial teflon catheters in that the taper of the catheter may be roughened or crimped if the material is not sufficiently strong to resist shearing forces during the passage through skin, subcutaneous tissue, and vessel wall. When this occurs a grating sensation is often detected as the needle is advanced into the artery. This complication calls for removal of the catheter, since it prevents the catheter from being advanced within the lumen of the artery. Furthermore the resulting unevenness of the catheter causes trauma (Fig. 46).

Finally, McNabb, Green, and Parker (17) have drawn attention to a potentially serious complication associated with the percutaneous placement of a Swan-Ganz catheter by the jugular route. In their case the catheter tip was presumed to have lodged in the wall of the carotid artery and although no harm came to the patient in this particular case, the complication is worth recording.

The most dramatic complication of central venous catheterization is perforation of the heart. This rare event is caused by displacement of the tip of the catheter and has been found to be on occasion as much as 8 cm with movement of the shoulder if the basilic vein is used for insertion of the catheter. Even if perforation does not occur, bruising of the caval wall is frequent. The subclavian route by providing greater stability avoids these complications (31). In another case percutaneous supraclavicular internal jugular vein catheterization led to puncture of the anterior wall of the ascending aorta in a patient with transposition of the great arteries (22). Lastly tension pneumothorax is a rare but serious complication of internal jugular cannulation (6).

Colvin, Savege, and Lewis (5) have described a case in which an infarct with some bleeding and oedematous reaction occurred around the end of a Swan-Ganz catheter that had been introduced with balloon deflated. The balloon was inflated only after the catheter tip had been firmly wedged and this produced local ischaemia. The point is made that the catheter must never be advanced into the pulmonary artery unless the balloon is inflated. Not unlike tracheal tubes,

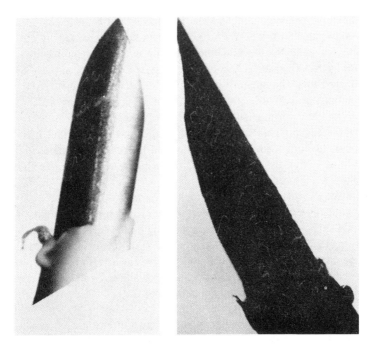

Figure 46 / Enlarged view of a catheter and cannulae showing sharp edges and projections.
From: Talmage (27); *courtesy: Anesthesia and Analgesia –Current Researches*

the tip of a Swan-Ganz catheter may become occluded because of overdistention of the cuff. Eccentric inflation may cause the tip to impinge on the vessel wall or to lie in the main stream. In either case erroneous pressure readings result (23). Balloons on wedge pressure catheters can cause, in common with tracheal tube cuffs, yet another complication, namely rupture while in use (2). These balloons are made of latex, a material which degrades rapidly when exposed to direct sunlight or high temperature and to certain atmospheric pollutants, such as hydrogen sulphide and nitrogen oxides. Suitable precautions in storing these articles should therefore be taken.

EPIDURAL CATHETERS

Epidural catheters for continuous epidural anaesthesia are inserted through a needle previously advanced into the epidural space. This being so, these catheters are subject to the same complications as all long catheters in that they may kink, bend, or break on removal because they have turned on themselves and become curled or knotted around a nerve root. Like other catheters inserted through a needle, they may be sheared off by the bevel if they are withdrawn while the needle is still in place. Apart from this, epidural catheters may fail for more specific reasons described by Abouleish (1). He found in three instances that catheters had kinked and had a hole at that site. The kink coincided with the skin level and was caused by the acute change of direction of almost 90 degrees where the catheter emerges from the skin. A kink, of course, renders injection of local anaesthetic impossible and a hole leads to loss of anaesthetic solution, either of which will cause failure of the block.

Not infrequently, although they fit the lumen of the Tuohy needle, epidural catheters fail to pass the eye of the needle. In other cases catheters were found to be not patent.

APPENDICES AND REFERENCES

Suggested anaesthetic check list

Any check list must be adapted to the facilities available in the Operating Room and to other local circumstances. Checks must be carried out in systematic fashion, preferably in a gas flow sequence from source to patient end of the delivery system.

The following is a suggested check sequence.

A. AVAILABILITY AND STATE OF READINESS OF EQUIPMENT AND AGENTS

1. *Gases*
   a Oxygen and Nitrous Oxide; Air (if available)
      i Pipeline supply turned on and pressurized;
      ii Cylinders full; no leaks from valve stem or yoke connection;
      iii Functioning Oxygen By-Pass.
   b Others: (if available and needed)
      Cylinders full; no leaks.
2. *Volatile anaesthetics*
   a Vaporizers on machine for desired agents;
   b Vaporizers filled;
   c Filling ports closed.
3. *Vacuum system*
   a System turned on;
   b Suction connected; no leaks;
   c Suction adequate at patient end of nozzle or catheter.
4. *Assembly*
   a Anaesthetic machine connected to gas sources;
   b Breathing circuit assembled and connected to common gas outlet;
   c Flammable agents removed if source of ignition present.

5. *Drugs*
   Adequate supply available of frequently used drugs.
6. *Routine equipment*
   a Laryngoscope
      i Blades of different shapes and sizes available;
      ii Light intensity adequate.
   b Tracheal Tubes and Airways of different sizes;
   c Stylet for tracheal tubes;
   d Magill forceps;
   e Syringes and Needles of all sizes;
   f Intravenous Solutions and Administration Sets.
7. *Special equipment*
   a Any required for a particular case (e.g. hypothermia blanket, etc.)
   b Location and state of readiness of
      i Defibrillators;
      ii Anti-hyperthermia equipment;
      iii Emergency drugs.

B. ANAESTHETIC MACHINE

1. *Flowmeters*
   a Position of rotameter bobbins at zero gas flow;
   b Gas flow through correct flowmeter;
   c Bobbin rotation at all levels of gas flow;
   d Back pressure test positive.
2. *Vaporizers*
   a Controls in "Off" position;
   b Back pressure test positive.
3. *Breathing circuit*
   a Circuit pressurized for leaks;
   b Non-rebreathing circuit: Competence of valves;
   c Circle absorption:
      i Proper filling of absorber;
      ii State of soda lime;
      iii Absence of leaks on pressurization;
      iv Valves present and competent.
   d Bain circuit:
      i Patency of inner tube;
      ii Test for proper connection.
4. *Scavenging system*
5. *Fail safe and alarms*

C. OTHER EQUIPMENT

1. *Masks*
   Proper fit to patient's face.
2. *Tracheal tube*
   a Patency of lumen;
   b Integrity of cuff.
3. *Connectors*
   Fit of tracheal tube connector to patient end of breathing circuit.
4 *Electrical equipment*
   Grounding and functioning.

Standards of interest to the anaesthetist

INTERNATIONAL STANDARDS ORGANIZATION (ISO)

Current Standards

ISO-32 (1977) Identification of Medical Gas Cylinders
ISO-R 407   Yoke Type Valve Connections for Small Gas Cylinders and for Anaesthetic and Resuscitation Purposes

In preparation

Advanced Stage:

Breathing Attachments for Anaesthetic Apparatus
     Part I. Conical Fittings and Adaptors
     Part II. Screw threaded Weight bearing Fittings
Continuous Flow Anaesthetic Machines
Tracheal Tubes
     Part I. General Requirements
     Part II. Oral and Nasal Tracheal Tubes — Magill Type
     Part III. Tracheal Tubes of the Murphy Type
     Part IV. Cole Tubes
Anaesthetic Reservoir Bags (Draft International Standard ISO/Dis 5362)
Oropharyngeal Airways (Draft International Standard ISO/Dis 5364)
Tracheostomy Tubes — Connections for Sizes of 6.0 mm and greater
Breathing Tubes used with Anaesthetic Apparatus (Draft International Standard ISO/Dis 5367)

Breathing Machines – Definitions, Connectors, Performance Evaluation, etc.
Anaesthesia Terminology (Draft International Standard ISO/Dis 4135)

In Working Draft Stage

Medical Gas Hose Assemblies
Keyed Filling Devices for Liquid Anaesthetics
Tracheostomy Tubes – Connnections for Sizes of 5.5 mm and less
Equipment for Prolonged Tracheal Intubation
Laryngoscopic Fittings – Detachable Blades
Laryngoscopic Fittings – Screw Threads for Miniature Lamps
Medical Gas Pipeline Systems

CANADA

Principal Standards Writing Body

Canadian Standards Association (CSA)

Current Standards

B 96 – 1965 Compressed Gas Cylinder Valve Outlet and Inlet Connections
  Piping
C 22.2 No. 125 – 1973 Electromedical Equipment
Z 32.1 – 1970 Code for Prevention of Explosions or Electric Shock in Hospital
  Operating Rooms.
Z 39 – 1959 Code for Marking of Portable Compressed Gas Containers to
  Identify the Material Contained
Z168.1 – 1970 Tracheal Tubes
Z168.2 – 1967 Endotracheal Tube Connectors and Adaptors
Z168.4 – 1975 Keyed Filling Devices Applied to Anaesthetic Equipment
Z180.1 – 1973 Purity of Compressed Air for Breathing Purposes
Z275.1 – 1971 Hyperbaric Facilities
Z305.1 – 1975 Non-Flammable Medical Gas Systems
Z305.4 – 1977 Qualification Requirements for Testing Agencies for Non-
  Flammable Medical Gas Piping Systems
AS 1169 – 1973 Rules for the Minimizing of Hazards Arising from the Use of
  Flammable Medical Agents and Non-Flammable Medical Gases (known as
  the SAA Medical Agents and Gases Safety Code)
AS 1715 Code of Practice for Respiratory Protection
AS 1716 Respiratory Protection Devices

In preparation

Z 32.1   Code for Prevention of Explosions or Electric Shock in Hospital
Operating Rooms
Z 32.2   Use of Electricity in Patient Care Areas
Z 32.4   Essential Electrical Systems for Hospitals
Z168.3   Continuous Flow Inhalation Anaesthetic Apparatus
Z168.5   Lung Ventilators
Z305.2   Connecting Assemblies for Medical Gas Systems
Z305.3   Pressure and Flow Control Devices for Medical Gas Systems
Z305.5   Recommended practices for Installers of Non-Flammable Medical Gas
Piping Systems
Z317.1   Plumbing, Drainage, and Other Piping Systems for Health Care
Facilities
Z317.2   Heating, Ventilating, and Air Conditioning for Health Care Facilities

AUSTRALIA

Principal Standards Writing Body

Standards Association of Australia (SAA)

Current Standards

AS T37-1966   Breathing Attachments for Anaesthetic Apparatus
AS CB4-1969   SAA Gas Cylinder Code, Supplement No. 1: Yoke Outlets for
Medical Gases.

Draft Standards

Respiratory Resuscitators, Resuscitator Units, Resuscitator Containers and
Resuscitator Kits.
Suction for Use in Hospitals

NEW ZEALAND

Principal Standards Writing Body

Standards Association of New Zealand (SANZ)

Current Standards

NZS 1304–1957 Medical Gas Cylinders and Anaesthetic Apparatus,
    Amendment No. 1
NZS 1361–1962 Anaesthetic Breathing Bags made of Anti-Static Rubber
NZS 1475–1959 Anaesthetic Airways, Amendment A:-1959
NZS 2107–1966 Breathing Machines for Medical Use, Amendment No. 1:-1966
NZS 2109–1966 Breathing Attachments for Anaesthetic Apparatus

UNITED KINGDOM

Principal Standards Writing Body

British Standards Institution (BSI)

Current Standards

Anaesthetic and Respiratory Equipment
B.S. 2927–1957 Anaesthetic Airways
B.S. 3353–1961 Anaesthetic Breathing Bags made of Anti-static Rubber
B.S. 3487–1962 Endotracheal Tubes
B.S. 3806–1964 Breathing Machines for Medical Use
B.S. 3849–1965 Breathing Attachments for Anaesthetic Apparatus
    Part I – 1968 Anaesthetic and Analgesic Machines – Anaesthetic Machines
        of the On-Demand Type Supplied with Nitrous Oxide and Oxygen from
        Separate Containers
    Part II – 1968 Anaesthetic and Analgesic Machines – Analgesic Machines
        of the On-Demand Type Supplied with Premixed Nitrous Oxide – Oxygen
        from a Single Container
B.S. 4494–1970 Humidifiers for Use with Breathing Machines

Surgical Suction Apparatus

B.S. 4199 Surgical Suction Apparatus
    Part I–1967 Electrically Operated Surgical Suction Apparatus of High
    Vacuum and High Air Displacement Type
    Part II–1968 Electrically Operated Surgical Suction Apparatus for
    Continuous Drainage
B.S. 5185–1975 Dental Vacuum Pipeline Services
B.S. 4957–1973 Medical Vacuum Pipeline Services for Use in Hospitals

Others

B.S. 1319–1955 Medical Gas Cylinders and Anaesthetic Apparatus
B.S. 2050–1961 Specification for Electrical Resistance of Conductive and Anti-static Products made from Flexible Polymeric Material
B.S. 3112–1959 General Purpose Trolleys for Anaesthetists' Use
B.S. 3574–1963 Storage of Vulcanized Rubber
B.S. 4843–1972 Sterile Intravenous Cannulae for Single Use

UNITED STATES OF AMERICA

Principal Standards Writing Body

American National Standards Institute (ANSI)

Current Standards

B57.1–1965 Pin-Index Safety System
Z79.1–1974 Tracheal Tubes and Cuffs
Z79.2–1976 Tracheal Tube Connectors and Adaptors
Z79.3–1974 Oropharyngeal Airways
Z79.4–1974 Anesthetic Reservoir Bags
Z79.5–1974 Murphy Tracheal Tubes
Z79.6–1975 Breathing Tubes
Z79.7–1976 Breathing Machines for Medical Use
Z86.1   Commodity Specification for Air, Grade F

In preparation

Z79.8 Minimum Performance and Safety Requirements for Components and Systems of Continuous-Flow Anesthesia Machines
Z79.X Terminology Related to Anesthesiology
Z79.X Tracheal Tubes and Cuffs for Prolonged Use
Z79.X Emergency Resuscitation
Z79.X Humidifiers and Nebulizers for Use with Breathing Machines
Z79.X Oxygen Analyzers
Z79.X Suction Catheters
Z79.X Antidisconnect System

DEVELOPED BY OTHER STANDARD SETTING GROUPS

ANSI/CGA V-1-1977   Compressed Gas Cylinder Valve Outlet and Inlet Connections

ANSI/NFPA 56B-1976 Respiratory Therapy

ANSI/NFPA 56D-1976 Hyperbaric Facilities

ANSI/NFPA 56F-1974 Nonflammable Medical Gas Systems (Revision submitted for ANSI approval)

STANDARDS NOT PUBLISHED AS AMERICAN NATIONAL STANDARDS

CGA V-5 Diameter Index Safety System Enlargement (CGA Docket 68-32-3)

CGA C-9 Color Coding of Medical Gas Cylinders (CGA Docket 71-16-6)

NFPA 56A Standard for Use of Inhalation Anesthetics

UL 544 Safety Standard for Medical and Dental Equipment

References

I INTRODUCTION

1 Brown, F.N., and Hilton, J.H.B. 1977. Inadvertence in anaesthesia leading to disaster. Seventy-sixth Annual Report, Canadian Medical Protective Association, pp. 15-18
2 Dorsch, J.A., and Dorsch, S.E. 1975. *Understanding Anesthesia Equipment: Construction, Care and Complications.* The Williams & Wilkins Co., Baltimore. pp. 67, 217
3 Dripps, R.D., Eckenhoff, J.E., and Vandam, L.D. 1972. *Introduction to Anesthesia. The Principles of Safe Practice.* (4th Ed.) W.B. Saunders Co., Philadelphia, pp. 61-62
4 Forrester, A.C. 1968. Anaesthetists-in-law. Proc. Roy. Soc. Med. 61(4): 409-416
5 Mainland, J. and Dudley, H. 1976. *Safety in the Operating Theatre.* Edward Arnold (Australia) Pty, Ltd., Melbourne, pp. 68-92
6 Nagle, D.R. Machines and men (Editorial) 1930. Brit. J. Anaesth., 7:97 Reprinted 1962 in Anesthesiology 23(1): 136-137
7 Ward, C.S. 1975. *Anaesthetic Equipment. Physical Principles and Maintenance.* Baillière Tyndall, London, pp. 84-86

II NON-FLAMMABLE MEDICAL GAS PIPELINE SYSTEMS

1 Anonymous. 1966. An accident in Edinburgh. The Lancet, Oct. 29
2 Anonymous. Medical Agents and Gases — Safety Code. Australian Standard AS 1169-1973, Part II
3 ANSI Standard Z86.1, Commodity Specification for Air, Grade F

4 CSA Standard Z305.1-1975, Non-Flammable Medical Gas Piping Systems. Canadian Standards Association, Rexdale, Ontario, Canada

5 Cundy, J.M. A safety feature for piped gas supplies (Corresp.). 1976. Anaesthesia 31(1): 109-110

6 Department of Health and Social Security. 1972. *Piped Medical Gases, Medical Compressed Air and Medical Vacuum Installation.* Hospital Technical Memorandum No. 22. H.M. Stationery Office, London

7 Dinnick, O.P. Personal communication

8 Eichhorn, J.H., Bancroft, M.L., Laasberg, L.H., Du Moulin, G.C. and Sauberman, A.J. 1977. Contamination of medical gas and water pipelines in Anesthesiology 46(4): 286-289

9 Feeley, T.W., and Hedley-White, J. 1976. Bulk oxygen and nitrous oxide delivery systems. Design and dangers. Anesthesiology 44(4): 301-305

10 Feeley, T.W., McClelland, K.J., and Malhotra, I.V. 1975. The hazards of bulk oxygen delivery systems. The Lancet, 1416-1418

11 Finlay, J., and Pelton, D.A. 1971. Needed: Error protection, hospitals. JAHA 45: 64-66

12 Hunter, A.R. 1977. Pipe-line accident (Corresp.). Brit. J. Anaesth. 49(3): 281-282

13 Hunter, A.R. 1977. Pipe-line accident (Corresp.). Anaesthesia 32(4): 383-384

14 IGC: Code of Practice for Supply Equipment and Pipelines Distributing Non-Flammable Gases and Vacuum Services for Medical Purposes. IGC Document 5/75/E

15 LeBourdois, E. 1974. Sudbury General inquest makes hospital history – nine deaths linked to cross-connection. Dimensions in Health Service 51(6): 10-12

16 Mazze, R.I. 1972. Therapeutic misadventures with oxygen delivery systems: The need for continuous in-line oxygen monitors. Anesth. & Analg. 51(5): 787-790

17 Morton, H.J.W. 1961. Maintenance of piped oxygen supplies (Corresp.). Anaesthesia, 16(2): 254

18 NFPA 50: Bulk Oxygen Systems, National Fire Protection Association, Boston, Mass., USA, 1974

19 NFPA Non-Flammable Medical Gas Systems. Code 56 F. National Fire Protection Association, Boston, Mass., USA

20 Nordland, R. and Ferrick, T. jr. 1977. Five die in mix-up at hospital, error undetected for six months. *Philadelphia Enquirer*, August 2

21 Pelton, D.A. 1969. Letters to the Editor. Can. Anaesth. Soc. J. 16(2): 173-174

22 Pelton, D.A. Personal communication

23 Sprague, D.H., and Archer, G.W. 1975. Intraoperative hypoxia from erroneously filled liquid oxygen reservoir. Anesthesiology 42(3): 360-362

24 Stodsky, B. 1949. To the Editor. Anesthesiology 10(3): 364
25 Wylie, W.D. 1975. There but for the grace of God . . Ann. R. Coll. Surg. Engl. 56(4): 171-180

III THE ANAESTHETIC MACHINE

General considerations

1 Austin, T.R. 1972. Metallic flanking: A further hazard of anaesthetic apparatus (Clinical Forum). Anaesthesia 27(1): 92-93
2 Dinnick, O.P. 1976. More problems with piped gases (Corresp.). Anaesthesia 31(6): 790-792
3 Dorsch, J.A., and Dorsch, S.E. 1975. *Understanding Anesthesia Equipment: Construction, Care and Complications.* The Williams and Wilkins Co., Baltimore. pp. 68-69
4 Eger, E.I., II, and Epstein, R.M. 1964. Hazards of anesthetic equipment. Anesthesiology 25(4): 490-504
5 Everett, G., Hornbein, T.F., and Allen, G.D. 1970. Hidden hazards of the McKesson Narmatic Anesthesia Machine (Clin. Wksp.). Anesthesiology 32(1): 73-75
6 Hutchinson, R.I. 1975. The accuracy and efficiency of general anaesthetic machines in dental practice. An investigation. Brit. Dent. J. 139(5): 187-189
7 Longmuir, J. and Craig, D.B. 1976. Misadventure with a Boyle's gas machine. (Letter to the Editor). Can. Anaesth. Soc. J. 23(6): 671-673
8 Mayer, A. 1973. Malfunction of anesthesia machines: a guide for maintenance. Anesth., Analg. 52(3): 376-382
9 Nainby-Luxmoore, R.C. 1967. Some hazards of dental gas machines. Anaesthesia 22(4): 545-555
10 Schweitzer, S.A. and Babarczy, A.J. 1976. An unexpected hazard of the Boyles machine. Anaesth. and Intens. Care 4(1): 72-73
11 Spoerel, W.E. The troubles with your anaesthesia machine. Unpublished
12 Youngman, H.R. 1958. Nitrous oxide by-pass (Corresp.). Brit. J. Anaesth. 30(1): 48
13 Youngman, H.R. 1958. Nitrous oxide bypass (Corresp.). Anaesthesia 13(2): 239

Compressed gas cylinders

1 Anonymous. 1945. Identification of gas cylinders (Medico-Legal). Brit. Med. J. 4393(1): 381
2 Anonymous. 1960. Commonwealth and foreign news. Australia Anaesthesia, 15(1): 101-102

3 Clutton-Brock, J. 1967. Two cases of poisoning by contamination of nitrous oxide with higher oxides of nitrogen during anaesthesia. Brit. J. Anaesth. 39(5): 388-392
4 Cole, P.V. 1964. Nitrous oxide and oxygen from a single cylinder. Anaesthesia 19(1): 3-11
5 Eger, E.I. II and Epstein, R.M. Hazards of Anesthetic Equipment. Anesthesiology, 25(4): 490-504 (Jul-Aug), 1964
6 Finch, J.S. A Report on a Possible Hazard of Gas Cylinder Tanks. (Corresp.) Anesthesiology, 33(4): 467 (Oct), 1970
7 Fox, J.W.C., and Fox, E.J. 1968. An unusual occurrence with a cyclopropane cylinder. Anesth., Analg. 47(5): 624-626
8 Lee, J.A., and Atkinson, R.S. 1968. *A Synopsis of Anaesthesia.* John Wright & Sons, Ltd., Bristol, 6th ed. p. 155
9 Mazze, R.I. 1972. Therapeutic misadventures with oxygen delivery systems: The need for continuous in-line monitors. Anesth., Analg. 51(5): 787-792
10 Rendell-Baker, L. Personal communication
11 Section on Anaesthetics. 1967. Impurities in nitrous oxide (Discussion). Proc. Roy. Soc. Med. 60: 1175-1180
12 Steward, D.J., and Sloan, I.A. 1973. Additional pin-indexing failures (Corresp.). Anesthesiology 39(3): 355
13 Thomas, G.J. 1955. Do you know? ASA Newsletter 19(8): 14-16
14 Tunstall, M.E. 1963. Pre-mixed gases (The Sections). Brit. Med. J., 2:240

Pin-index safety system

1 Anonymous. 1975 (Editorial). Can. Anaesth. Soc. J. 22(2): 123
2 Compressed Gas Association, Inc. 1975. Compressed gas cylinder valve outlet and inlet connections. Proposed revisions. July
3 Edwards, G., Morton, H.J.V., Pask. E.A., and Wylie, W.D. 1956. Deaths associated with anaesthesia: A report of 1000 cases. Anaesthesia 11(3): 194-220
4 Harroun, P., and Hathaway, H.R. 1944. An aid in preventing the interchange of cylinders during the administration of anesthetic gases (Current Comment and Case Reports). Anesthesiology, 5(5): 526-528
5 Hogg, C.E. 1973. Pin-indexing failures (Clin. Wksp.). Anesthesiology 38(1): 85-87
6 Lundy, J.S., and Seldon, T.H. 1940. Device to prevent gas mix-ups. Mod. Med. 55: 96, 1940 (abstracted in Anesthesiology 2(2): 236
7 MacIntosh, R.R. 1949. Deaths under anaesthetics. Brit. J. Anaesth. 21(3): 107-136

8 Minuck, M. 1967. Death in the operating room. Can. Anaesth. Soc. J. 14(3): 197
9 Rawstron, R.E., and McNeil, T.D. Pin-index system (Corresp.). 1962. Brit. J. Anaesth. 34(8): 591-592
10 Steward, D.J., and Sloan, I.A. 1973. Additional pin-indexing failures (Corresp.). Anesthesiology 39(3): 355
11 White, C.W., jr. 1970. ASA and the standardization of anesthesia equipment (Guest Editorial). ASA Newsletter 34(1): 2
12 Wolff, J.D., Lionarons, H.B., and Mesdag, M.J. 1970. A failure of the pin-index system of anesthetic gas tube connections. A case report. Arch. Chir. Neerl. 22(4): 243-245

Pressure regulators

1 Anonymous. 1952. Explosion hazards (Morbidity Conference). Brit. J. Anaesth. 24(4): 300-302
2 Dinnick, O.P. Personal communication
3 Hamelberg, W., Maffey, J.S., and Band, W.E. 1961. Nitrous oxide impurities. Anesth. Analg. 40(4): 408-411
4 Kalra, A.N., and Doughty, A.G. 1963. The wrong gas (corresp.). Anaesthesia 18(2): 234-236

Flowmeters

1 Battig, C.G. 1972. Unusual failure of an oxygen flowmeter. Anesthesiology 37(5): 561-562
2 Bishop, C., Levick, C.H., and Hodgson, C. 1967. A design fault in the Boyle apparatus (Corresp.). Brit. J. Anaesth. 39(11) 908
3 Calverley, R.K. 1971. A safety feature for anaesthetic machines – touch identification of oxygen flow control. Can. Anaesth. Soc. J. 18(2): 225-229
4 Chadwick, D.A. 1974. Transposition of rotameter tubes (Corresp.). Anesthesiology 40(1): 102
5 Clutton-Brock, J. 1972. Static electricity and rotameters. Brit. J. Anaesth. 44(1): 86-90
6 Clutton-Brock, J. 1972. Static electricity and rotameters (Corresp.). Brit. J. Anaesth. 44(4): 415
7 Dinnick, O.P. 1963. Accidental severe hypercarbia during anaesthesia (Corresp.). Brit. J. Anaesth. 40(1): 36
8 Dinnick, O.P. Personal communication
9 Edwards, G., Morton, H.J.V., Pask, E.A., and Wylie, W.D. 1956. Deaths associated with anaesthesia: a report of 1000 Cases. Anaesthesia 11(3): 194-220

10 Eger, E.L. II, Hylton, R.R., Irwin, R.H., and Guadagni, N. 1963. Anesthetic flowmeter sequence – a cause for hypoxia (Current Comment). Anesthesiology 24(3): 396-397

11 Eger, E.I. II, and Epstein, R.M. 1964. Hazards of anesthetic equipment. Anesthesiology 25(4): 490-504

12 Gupta, B.L., and Varshneya, A.K. 1975. Anaesthetic accident caused by unusual leakage of rotameter (Corresp.). Brit. J. Anaesth. 47(7): 805

13 Katz, D. 1968. Recurring cyanosis of intermittent mechanical origin in anesthetized patients. Anesth. Analg. 47(3): 233-237

14 Katz, D. 1969. Increasing the safety of anesthesia machines. I. Further modification of the Draeger machine. II. Considerations for the standardization of certain basic components. Anesth. Analg. 48(2): 242-245

15 Kelley, J.M., and Gabel, R.A. 1970. The improperly calibrated flowmeter – another hazard (Corresp.). Anesthesiology 33(4): 467-468

16 Liew, R.P.C. 1973. Oxygen loss down the third flowmeter (Corresp.). Anaesthesia 28(5): 579

17 Liew, P.C., and Garmendran, A. 1973. Oxygen failure: A potential danger with air-flowmeters in anaesthetic machine with remote controlled needle valves. Brit. J. Anaesth. 45(4): 1165-1168

18 Lomanto, C., and Leeming, M. 1970. A safety signal for detection of excessive anesthetic gas flows (Clin. Wksp.). Anesthesiology 33(6): 663-664

19 Mazze, R.I. 1972. Therapeutic misadventures with oxygen delivery systems: The need for continuous in-line monitors. Anesth. Analg. 51(5): 787-792

20 Muliyil, J.A. 1976. Anaesthetic accident caused by unusual leakage of rotameter (Corresp.). Brit. J. Anaesth. 48(5): 499

21 Prickett, G.L. 1972. A potential danger (Corresp.). Brit. J. Anaesth. 44(12): 1335

22 Prys-Roberts, C., Smith, W.D.A., and Nunn, J.F. 1967. Accidental severe hypercapnia during anaesthesia. Brit. J. Anaesth. 39(3): 257-267

23 Rees, D.F. 1972. Static electricity and rotameters (Corresp.). Brit. J. Anaesth. 44(4): 415

24 Rendell-Baker, L. 1976. Some gas machine hazards and their elimination. Anesth. Analg. 55(1): 26-33

25 Rendell-Baker, L. 1976. Anaesthetic accident caused by unusual leakage of rotameter (Corresp.). Brit. J. Anaesth. 48(5): 500

26 Richardson, J.C. 1972. A potential danger (Corresp.). Brit. J. Anaesth. 44(6): 610

27 Ross, E.D.T. 1968. Accidental hypercapnia and rotameter bobbins (Corresp.). Brit. J. Anaesth. 40(1): 45

28 Sadove, M.S., Thomason, R.D., Thomason, C.L., and Ries, M. 1976. An Evaluation of flowmeters. Am. Assoc. Nurse Anesth. J. 44(2): 162-165
39 Slater, E.M. 1974. Transposition of rotameter bobbins (Corresp.). Anesthesiology 41(1): 101
30 Spoerel, W.E. The troubles with your anaesthesia machine. Unpublished
31 Trubuhovich, R.V. 1967. Carbon dioxide cylinders on anaesthetic machines (Corresp.). Brit. J. Anaesth. 39(7): 607-608
32 Varshney, J.P. 1976. Anaesthetic accident caused by unusual leakage of rotameter (Corresp.). Brit. J. Anaesth. 48(5): 499-500

Vaporizers

1 Adner, M., and Hallen, B. 1965. Reliability of halothane vaporizers. Acta Anaesth. Scandin. 9(4): 233-239
2 Canadian Standards Association. Keyed filling devices applied to anaesthetic equipment. CSA Standard Z 168.4-1975
3 Chun, L., and Karp, M. 1964. Accidental use of trichlorethylene (Trilene® Trimar® in a closed system. Case history #39. Anesth. Analg. 43(6): 740-743
4 Cohen, D.D., and Groveman, J.E. 1966. "Explosion" in an anesthesia vaporizer (Current Comment). Anesthesiology 27(3): 331
5 De Guzman, C.M., and Cascorbi, H.F. 1972. An unusual hazard of methoxyflurane (Clin. Wksp.). Anesthesiology 36(3): 305
6 Eger, E.I. II, 1963. Pressure effect on the vernitrol vaporizer (Corresp.). Anesthesiology 24(5): 742
7 Eldrup-Jorgensen, S., and Sprissler, G.T. 1977. Gas leaks in anesthesia machines (Corresp.). Anesthesiology 46(6): 439
8 Gabel, R.A., and Danielsen, J.B. 1971. Backflow of liquid halothane into a flowmeter (Corresp.). Anesthesiology 34(5): 492-493
9 Gordh, T., Hallen, B., Okmian, L., Wahlin, A., and Stern, B. 1964. The Concentration of halothane by the combined use of fluotec vaporizer and Engström respirator. Acta Anaesth. Scandin. 8(2): 97-105
10 Gorgerino, F., Gazzano, A.M., and Vassoney, G. 1966. Anesthesia problems at high altitude: Halothane vaporization. Proceedings 1 of the Second European Congress of Anaesthesiology, Copenhagen, Aug. 8-13, 1966. Acta Anaesth. Scandin. Suppl. XXIII: 491-494
11 Greenhow, D.E., and Barth, R.L. 1973. Oxygen flushing delivers anesthetic vapor — A hazard with a new machine (Corresp.). Anesthesiology 38(4): 409-410
12 Haldemann, G., Hossli, G., and Schaer, H. 1973. Über die Verdampfungsleistung des Oxford Miniature Vaporizer (OMV) für Halothane. (The Efficacy of

the Oxford Miniature Vaporizer for Halothane.) Der Anaesthesist 22(8): 339-344

13 Hall, J.M., Hellewell, J., Fisher, E.L., Burns, T.H.S., and Fuzzey, G.J.J. 1966. A test of two types of halothane vaporizers. Brit. J. Anaesth. 38(6): 494-497

14 Hill, D.W. 1958. Halothane concentrations with Fluotec vaporizer. Brit. J. Anaesth. 30(12): 563-567

15 Hill, D.W., and Lowe, H.J. 1962. Comparison of concentration of halothane in closed and semi-closed circuits during controlled ventilation. Anesthesiology 23(3): 291-298

16 Kapfhammer, V., and Atabas, A. 1965. Der Fluotec Mark II mit angebautem Druckausgleichventil. (The Fluotec Mark II with incorporated pressure-equilibrating valve.) Der Anaesthesist 14(9): 257-259

17 Keenan, Major R.L. 1963. Prevention of increased pressures in anesthetic vaporizers with a unidirectional valve (Current Comment). Anesthesiology 24(5): 732-734

18 Keet, J.E., Valentine, G.W., and Riccio, J.S. 1963. An arrangement to prevent pressure effect on the Vernitrol vaporizer (Current Corresp.). Anesthesiology 24(5): 734-737

19 Keet, J.E., Valentine, G.W., and Riccio, J.S. 1963. An arrangement to prevent pressure effect on the Vernitrol vaporizer (Corresp.). Anesthesiology 24(5): 742-743

20 Kopriva, C.J., and Lowenstein, E. 1969. An anesthetic accident: Cardiovascular collapse from liquid halothane delivery (Clin. Wksp.) Anesthesiology 30(2): 246-247

21 Larsen, E.R. 1972. Foaming in halogenated anesthetics – the Chemistry of modern inhalation anesthetics. In *Modern Inhalation Anesthetics*, ed. Chenoweth, M.B. Springer Verlag, New York, p. 29

22 Marks, W.E., and Bullard, J.R. 1976. Another hazard of free-standing vaporizers. Increased anesthetic concentration with reversed flow of vaporizing gas (Clin. Report). Anesthesiology 45(4): 445-446

23 McBurney, R. Letter to the Editor. 1977. Can. Anaesth. Soc. J. 24(3): 417-418

24 Morgan, M., and Lumley, J. 1968. Reliability of halothane vaporizers. Fluotec MK.2 and Halothane 4(MIE). Anaesthesia 23(3): 440-445

25 Morgan, M., and Lumley, J. Letter to the Editor. 1970. Can Anaesth. Soc. J. 17(5): 544

26 Mulroy, M., Ham, J., and Eger, E.I. II, 1976. Inflowing gas leak, a potential source of hypoxia. Anesthesiology 45(1): 102-104

27 Munson, Major W.M. 1965. Cardiac arrest: Hazard of tipping a vaporizer (Current Comment). Anesthesiology 26(2): 235

28 Murray, W.J., and Fleming, P. 1972. Fluotec MK .2 halothane output: Non-linearity from off to 0.5 percent dial setting (Clin. Wksp.). Anesthesiology 36(2): 180-181

29 Murray, W.J., Zsigmond, E.K., and Fleming, P. 1973. Contamination of in-series vaporizers with halothane-methoxyflurane (Clin. Wksp.). Anesthesiology 38(5): 487-490

30 Noble, W.H. Accuracy of halothane vaporizers in clinical use. 1970. Can. Anaesth. Soc. J. 17(2): 135-144

31 Paull, J.D., and Sleeman, V.W. 1972. An anaesthetic hazard (Corresp.). Brit. J. Anaesth. 43(12): 1202

32 Rendell-Baker, L. 1976. Some gas machine hazards and their elimination. Anesth. Analg. 55(1): 26-33

33 Safar, P., and Galla, S.J. 1962. Overdose with Ohio halothane vaporizer (Case Report). Anesthesiology 23(5): 715-716

34 Schreiber, P. 1972. Anaesthesia Equipment. Performance, Classification and Safety. Springer-Verlag, Berlin, Heidelberg, New York, p. 56

35 Sweatman, F. 1973. Foaming of methoxyflurane contaminated with silicone. Anesthesiology 38(4): 407

36 Tammisto, T. 1966. Measurements of concentrations of halothane with Gardner Universal vaporizers. Proceedings 1 of the Second European Congress of Anaesthesiology, Copenhagen, Aug. 8-13, 1966. Acta Anaesth. Scandin., Suppl. XXIII: 507-512

37 Weis, K.H., and Schreiber, P. 1965. Konzentrations Messungen mit dem Gardner-Universal-Verdampfer. (Measurement of concentrations delivered by the Gardner Universal Vaporizer). Der Anaesthesist 14(10): 289-293

38 Wickett, R.E., Jenkins, L.C., and Root, L.S. 1974. Downstream contamination of in-series vaporizers. Can. Anaesth. Soc. J. 21(1): 114-116

Fail-safe systems

1 Adler, L., and Burn, N. 1957. A warning device for failure of the oxygen supply (Apparatus). Anaesthesia 22(1): 156-159

2 Anonymous. 1962. Oxygen and the anesthesia machine (Clinical Anesthesia Conference). N.Y. State J. Med. 62(17): 2845-2846

3 Austin, T.R. 1971. warning device for the Flutoc Mark II and III (Clinical Forum). Anaesthesia 26(3): 368

4 Boba, A. 1975. The fallacy of failsafes (Corresp.). Anesthesiology 43(1): 131-132

5 Cooke, M., and Waine, T.E. 1967. Oxygen warning device connected directly to the oxygen cylinder (Apparatus). Anaesthesia 22(3): 487-488

6 Craig, D.B., and Longmuir, J. 1971. An unusual failure of an oxygen fail-safe device. Can. Anaesth. Soc. J. 18(5): 576-577

7 Davenport, H.T., and Wright, B.M. 1974. Simple oxygen-failure safety device (New Inventions). Brit. Med. J. III (5930): 570-571

8 Davenport, H.T., and Wright, B.M. 1974. Simple oxygen-failure safety device (Corresp.). Brit. Med. J. IV (5941): 407

9 Dorsch, J.A., and Dorsch, S.E. 1975. *Understanding Anesthesia Equipment: Construction, Care and Complications.* The Williams & Wilkins Company, Baltimore

10 Epstein, R.M., Rackow, H., Lee, A.S.J., and Papper, E.M. 1962. Prevention of accidental breathing of anoxic gas mixtures during anesthesia. Anesthesiology 23(1): 1-4

11 Esplen, J.R. 1956. A device giving warning of impending failure of the nitrous oxide or oxygen supply. Brit. J. Anaesth. 28(5): 226-227

12 Falkner Hill, E. 1956. Another warning device. Brit. J. Anaesth. 28(5): 228-229

13 Fraser-Jones, J., Jenkins, A.V., and Thomas, E. 1965. Intermittent positive pressure respirators and the 'Bosun' oxygen warning device (Corresp.). Anesthesia 20(1): 95-96

14 Grogono, A.W. 1965. Warning device for oxygen cylinders (New Inventions). Lancet 1 (7377): 144-145

15 Hurter, D.G., and Williams, D. 1964. The Bosun device (Corresp.). Lancet (2): 480

16 Lucas, B.G.B. 1967. A 'fail safe' oxygen device (New Appliances). Brit. Med. J. 1(5539): 551

17 Matteo, R.S., Gissen, A., and Lee, A.St.J. 1969. Safety in the Use of nitrous oxide (Techn. Notes). Anesthesiology 31(4): 361-369

18 Parfitt, R. 1973. Anaesthetic safety devices (Corresp.). Brit. Med. J., III (5881): 635

19 Robinson, J.S. 1974. Simple oxygen-failure safety device (Corresp.). Brit. Med. J. IV (5941): 407

20 Rosen, M., and Hillard, E.K. 1971. Oxygen fail-safe device for an anesthetic apparatus. Brit. J. Anaesth. 43(1): 103-106

21 Sawa, T., and Ikezomo, E. 1970. A respirator alarm for general use (Clin. Wksp.). Anesthesiology 33(6): 658-661

22 Scurlock, J.E. 1975. More failsafe failsafes (Clin. Reports). Anesthesiology 42(2): 226-228

23 Sladen, A., and Kelley, C. 1970. Fail-safe apneic control in the Bird venti-lator (Clin- Wksp.). Anesthesiology 33(1): 111-112

24 Ward, C.S. 1968. Oxygen warning device. Brit. J. Anaesth. 40(11): 907-908

25 Ward, C.S. 1975. *Anaesthetic Equipment: Physical Principles and Maintenance.* Bailliere Tindall, London

26 Wilson, A. Murray. 1965. Warning devices on anaesthetic apparatus. With a description of a new device. Anaesthesia 20(4): 403-407

27 Wright, B.M. 1976. Memorandum on oxygen supply pressure failure warning and protection devices (Corresp.). Anaesthesia 31(4): 568-569

IV THE BREATHING SYSTEM

General considerations

1 Arens, J.F. 1971. A hazard in the use of an Ayre T-piece. Anesth. Analg. 50(6): 943-946

2 Brière, C., Patoine, J.C., and Audet, R. 1974. Inaccurate ventrimetry by fresh gas inlet position. Can. Anaesth. Soc. J. 21(1): 117-119

3 Cottrell, J.E., Bernhard, W., and Turndorf, H. 1976. Hazards of disposable rebreathing circuits (Brief reports). Anesth. Analg. 55(5): 743-744

4 Cottrell, J.E., Chalon, J., and Turndorf, H. 1977. Faulty anesthetic circuits: a source of environmental pollution in the operating room. Anesth. Analg. 56(3): 359-362

5 Debban, D.G., Capt., and Bedford, R.F., Major. 1975. Overdistention of the rebreathing bag, a hazardous test for circle-system integrity (Clin. Reports). Anesthesiology 42(3): 365-366

6 Dinnick, O.P. 1973. Hazards of respiratory circuits. (Symposium on 'Hazards in the Operating Theatre'). Ann. Roy. Coll. Surg. Engl. 52: 349-354

7 Dorsch, J.A., and Dorsch, S.E. 1975. *Understanding Anesthesia Equipment: Construction, Care and Complications.* The Williams and Wilkins Co., Baltimore, p. 68

8 Dorsch, S.E. 1975. ASA Committee on Mechanical Equipment Issues Equipment Alert. ASA Newsletter 39(1): 4

9 Edwards, G., Morton, H.J.V., Pask, E.A., and Wylie, W.D. 1956. Deaths Associated with anaesthesia: A report of 1000 cases. Anaesthesia 11(3): 194-220

10 Page, J. 1977. Testing for leaks (Corresp.) Anaesthesia 32(7): 673

11 Ribak, Major B. 1975. Reducing the soda-lime hazard (Corresp.). Anesthesiology 43(2): 277

12 Witcher, C., Piziali, R., Sher, R., and Moffat, R.J. 1975. Development and evaluation of methods for the elimination of waste anesthetic gases and vapors in hospitals. Cincinatti, Ohio. U.S. Dept. of Health, Education and Welfare, Public Health Service, Center for Disease Control, Nat. Institute for Occupational Safety and Health, Division of Field Studies and Clinical Investigation, pp. VI/1-4

Breathing bags, tubes, and bacterial filters

1 Berry, F.A., Jr., and Eastwood, D.W. 1967. Serious defects in 'simple' equipment. Anesthesiology 28(2): 471
2 Breen, M. 1975. Letter to the Editor. Can. Anaesth. Soc. J. 22(2): 247
3 Cozanitis, D.A., and Takkunen, O. 1971. Aneurysm of ventilator tubing. A warning (Apparatus). Anaesthesia 26(2): 235-236
4 Foëx, P. and Crampton Smith, A. 1977. A test for co-axial circuits. Anaesthesia 32(3): 294
5 Hannalah, R., and Rosales, J.K. 1974. A hazard connected with re-use of the Bain's circuit. A case report. Can. Anaesth. Soc. J. 21(5): 511-513
6 Kopman, A.F., and Glaser, L. 1976. Obstruction of bacterial filters by edema fluid (Clin. Reports). Anesthesiology 44(2): 169-170
7 Lynch, C.G.M. 1976. The tail of a bag: A hazard (Corresp.). Anaesthesia 31(6): 803-804
8 Mansell, W.H. 1976. Bain circuit: 'The hazard of the hidden tube.' Can. Anaesth. Soc. J. 23(2): 227
9 Parmley, J.B., Tahir, A.H., Dascomb, H.E., and Adriani, J. 1972. Disposable versus reusable rebreathing circuits: Advantages, disadvantages, hazards and bacteriologic studies. Anesth. Analg. 51(6): 888-894
10 Paterson, J.G., and Vanhooydonk, V. 1975. A hazard associated with improper connection of the Bain breathing circuit. Can. Anaesth. Soc. J. 22(3): 373-377
11 Pethick, S.L. 1975. Letter to the Editor. Can. Anaesth. Soc. J. 22(1): 115
12 Salt, R. 1977. A test for co-axial circuits (Corresp.) Anaesthesia 32(7): 675-676
13 Sugg, B.R. 1977. Defective and misused co-axial circuits. Misuse of co-axial circuits. Anaesthesia 32(3): 293-294
14 Wildsmith, J.A.W., and Grubb, D.J. 1977. Defective and misused co-axial circuits. Faulty co-axial circuits. Anaesthesia 32(3): 293

Carbon dioxide absorbers

1 Beyermann-Urbig, G. 1964. Eine eigenartige technische Störung während einer Anaesthesie (Fehler und Gefahren). (A unique technical difficulty during anaesthesia) Der Anaesthesist, 13(10): 345
2 Danielson, H. 1958. Canisters with shunt valve arm (Corresp.). Anesthesiology 19(4): 564
3 Edwards, G., Morton, H.J.V., Pask, E.A., and Wylie, W.D. 1956. Deaths associated with anaesthesia: A report of 1000 cases. Anaesthesia 11(3): 194-220

4 Gartrell, P. 1975. Design of Boyle absorber (Corresp.). Anaesth. Intens. Care 3(2): 160-161
5 Mainland, J.F. 1975. Design of Boyle absorber (Corresp.). Anaesth. Intens. Care 3(2): 161
6 Marcus, P.S., and Ogden, A.E. 1959. Complications encountered by Anesthesiologists. Anesth. Analg. 38(6): 451-460
7 Nealon, T.F., Chase, H.F., and Gibbon, J.H. 1958. Factors influencing carbon dioxide absorption during anesthesia. Anesthesiology 19(1): 75-81
8 Owen, S.B. 1956. Defective carbon dioxide absorption in anesthetic machine (Current Comment). Anesthesiology 17(6): 829-830
9 Ringrose, N.H. 1974. Design of the Boyle absorber. Anaesth. Intens. Care 2(3): 269-271
10 Whitten, M.P., and Wise, C.C. 1972. Design faults in commonly used carbon dioxide absorbers. Brit. J. Anaesth. 44(5): 535-537

Valves

1 Anonymous. 1965. Misuse of relaxants in iatrogenic respiratory obstruction (Clinical Anesthesia Conference). N.Y. State J. Med. 65(6): 793-794
2 Anonymous. 1969. Hazards to avoid when using equipment with valved Y-piece ASA Newsletter 33(9): 7
3 Anonymous. 1975. Inquest into the death of Reta McVeety (Verdict of Coroner's Jury). Peel County Courthouse, Brampton, Ont., 12 Nov.
4 Askrog, V., and Elb, S. 1966. Experiments with non-rebreathing anesthesia systems during controlled ventilation. Anesth. Analg. 45(3): 348-351
5 Clementsen, H.J., Wolff, G., and Hugin, W. 1964. Die Funktionsveränderungen des EMO Inhalers durch Kombination mit dem Ambu-Beatmungsbeutel und Ruben-Ventil (The changes in function of the EMO inhaler when combined with the Ambu bag and Ruben valve). Der Anaesthesist 13(1): 15-21
6 Dean, H.N., Capt., Parsons, D.E., and Raphaely, R.C. 1971. Case Report: Bilateral tension pneumothorax from mechanical failure of anesthesia machine due to misplaced expiratory valve. Anesth. Analg. 50(2): 195-198
7 Ditzler, J. 1970. Checking anesthesia machines (Corresp.). Anesthesiology 32(1): 87
8 Doğu, T.S., and Davis, H.S. 1970. Hazards of inadvertently opposed valves (Corresp.) Anesthesiology 33(1): 122-123
9 Holland, R. 1970. Special committee investigating deaths under anaesthesia: Memorandum on the dangers of non-breathing valves (Corresp.). Med. J. Australia 2(1): 46-47
10 Lin, M.K. 1969. Severe hypercarbia due to the functional failure of swivel Y valves during anesthesia. Jap. J. Anesth. 18: 879-883

11 Meyer, M. 1966. Uber die Effektivität des Ruben-Ventils bei Spontanatmung und druckpositiver Inspiration (The effectiveness of the Ruben Valve during Spontaneous Respiration and Positive Pressure Inspiration). Der Anaesthesist 15(6): 189-193

12 Norry, H.T. 1972. A pressure limiting valve for anaesthetic and respirator circuits. Can. Anaesth. Soc. J. 19(5): 583-588

13 Rendell-Baker, L. 1969. Another close call with crossed valves (Corresp.). Anesthesiology 31(2): 194-195

14 Ruben, H. 1966. Uber die effectivität des Ruben-Ventils bei Spontanatmung und druckpositiver Inspiration (The effectiveness of the Ruben valve during spontaneous respiration and positive pressure inspiration). Der Anaesthesist 15(8): 270-271

15 Russell, W.J. and Drew, S.A. 1977. A potential hazard with the inspiratory valve of a circle system. Anaesth. & Int. Care 5(3): 269-271

16 Rusz, T., and Duncalf, D. 1970. A safe controlled pop-off valve (Clin. Wksp.) Anesthesiology 33(4): 459-461

17 Vogel, H., Hakim, A., and Pflüger, H. 1969. Rückatmung bei Verwendung von Ruben-Ventilen (Rebreathing with the use of the Ruben valve). Der Anaesthesist 18(8): 247-249

18 White, C.W., Jr. 1970. ASA and the standardization of anesthesia equipment (Guest Editorial). ASA Newsletter 34(1): 2

19 White, C.W., Jr. 1970. Hazards of the valved Y-piece (Corresp.). Anesthesiology 32(6): 567

Connectors and adaptors

1 Ballantyne, R.I.W., and Jackson, I. 1954. Anaesthesia for neurosurgical operations. Anaesthesia 9(1): 4-12

2 Beves, P.H. 1960. An Anaesthetic hazard (Corresp.). Brit. J. Anaesth. 32(9): 447

3 Collier, C.B. 1977. Blockage of endotracheal tube connectors (Corresp.). Anaesth. Intens. Care, 5(1): 85-86

4 Dolan, P.F. 1976. A simple safety device (Corresp.). Brit. J. Anaesth. 48(5): 499

5 Forrester, A.C. 1969. Mishaps in anaesthesia. Anaesthesia 14(4): 388-399

6 Galway, J.E. 1972. Airway obstruction (Corresp.). Anaesthesia 27(1): 102-103

7 Haley, F.C. 1975. Correspondence Can. Anaesth. Soc. J. 22(5): 628-629

8 Hewer, C.L. 1956. Asphyxia due to faulty apparatus (Corresp.). Brit. Med. J. 2: 766-767

9 Marshall, T., and Lewis, J.M. 1968. Fault in Endotracheal adaptor (Corresp.). Brit. J. Anaesth. 40(5): 393

10 Masson, A.H.B. 1960. An anaesthetic hazard (Corresp.). Brit. J. Anaesth. 32(7): 342-343

11 McKinley, A.C. 1977. Occlusion of an endotracheal tube connector (Corresp.). Anesthesiology 47(5): 480

12 McLellan, I. 1975. Blockage of tracheal connectors with K-Y jelly (Corresp.). Anaesthesia 30(3): 413-416

13 Osterud, A. 1974. Dangerous fault in disposable connector for orotracheal tube (Corresp.). Brit. J. Anaesth. 46(12): 952

14 Robbie, D.S., and Pearce, D.J. 1959. Some dangers of armoured tubes. Anaesthesia 14(4): 379-385

15 Rollason, W.N. 1956. Asphyxia due to faulty apparatus (Corresp.). Brit. Med. J. 2: 658

16 Ross, E.D.T. 1974. Misuse of the plug of Cobb's suction union (Apparatus). Anaesthesia 29(1): 66-68

17 Shaw, E.A. 1971. Airway obstruction (Clinical Forum). Anaesthesia 26(3): 368-3

18 Singh, C.V. 1977. Bizarre airway obstruction (Corresp.). Anaesthesia 32(8): 812-813

19 Star, E.G. 1975. A simple safety device (Corresp.). Brit. J. Anaesth. 47(9): 1034

20 Stark, D.D.C. 1976. Endotracheal tube obstruction (Corresp.). Anesthesiologist 45(4): 467-468

Scavenging devices

1 Best, D.W.S. 1971. A simple inexpensive system for the removal of excess anaesthetic vapours. Can. Anaesth. Soc. J. 18(3): 333-338

2 Boyd, C.H. 1972. Do-it-yourself venting appliance for use with a popular expiratory valve. Brit. J. Anaesth. 44(9): 992

3 Bruce, D.L., and Bach, M.J. 1975. Psychological studies of human performance as affected by traces of enflurane and nitrous oxide. Anesthesiology 42(2): 194-196

4 Bruce, D.L., Bach, M.J., and Arbit, J. 1974. Trace Anaesthetic effects on perceptual, cognitive and motor skills. Anesthesiology 40(5): 453-458

5 Bullough, J. 1954. Anaesthetic explosions, prevention by withdrawal methods. Lancet 1: 798-801

6 Cameron, H. 1970. Pollution control in the operating room, a simple device for the removal of expired anaesthesia vapours. Can. Anaesth. Soc. J. 17(5): 535-539

7 Carson, W., Ma, W.Y.L., and Legg, R.C. 1964. Air conditioning in hospitals — with special reference to operating theatres. Hosp. Engr. 18: 40

8 Cohen, E.N., Bellville, J.W., and Brown, B.W. 1971. Anaesthesia, pregnancy and miscarriage, a study of operating room nurses and anaesthetists. Anesthesiology 35(4): 343-347

9 Cohen, E.N., Brown, B.W., Bruce, D.L., Cascorbi, H.F., Corbett, T.H., Jones, T., and Whitcher, C.E. 1974. Occupational disease among operating room personnel, a national study. Anesthesiology 41(4): 321-340

10 Davies, G., and Tarnawsky, M. 1976. Letters to the Editor. Can. Anaesth. Soc. J. 230(2): 228

11 Enderby, G.E.H. 1972. Gas exhaust valve. Anaesthesia 27(3): 334-337

12 Evans-Prosser, C.D.G. 1972. A circuit to reduce the inhalation of gases by anaesthetists. Brit. J. Anaesth. 44(4): 412

13 Jørgenson, S. 1973. Scavenging systems on anaesthetic machines. Lancet 1: 672

14 Lecky, J.H., Springstead, J.M., and Neufeld, G.R. *In-House Manual for the Control of Anaesthetic Gas Contamination in the Operating Room.* University of Pennsylvania, Department of Anesthesia.

15 McInnes, I.C., and Goldwater, H.L. 1972. Gas removal systems for commonly used circuits. Anaesthesia 27(3): 340-347

16 Parbrook, G.D., and Monk, I.B. 1975. An expired gas collection and disposal system. Brit. J. Anaesth. 47(11): 1185-1193

17 Price, M., and McKeever, R. 1970. Anaesthetic anti-pollution device. Can. Anaesth. Soc. J. 17(5): 540

18 Scott, J.K. Unpublished

19 Sharock, N.E., and Leith, D.E. 1977. Potential pulmonary barotrauma, when venting anaesthetic gases to suction. Anesthesiology 46(2): 152-154

20 Sniper, W., and Murchison, A.G. 1972. A simple anaesthetic expiration flue, and its functional analysis. Brit. J. Anaesth. 44(11): 1222

21 Steward, D.J. 1972. An anti-pollution device for use with the Jackson Rees modification of Ayre's T-piece. Can. Anaesth. Soc. J. 19(6): 670-671

22 Vaisman, A.I. 1967. Working conditions in surgery, and their effects on the health of anaesthesiologists. Eksp. Khir. Anest. 3: 44

23 Vaughan, R.S., Mapleson, W.W., and Mushin, W.W. 1973. Prevention of pollution of operating theatres with halothane vapour by absorption with activated charcoal. Brit. Med. J. 1: 727-729

24 Yeakel, A.E. 1970. A device for elimination overflow anaesthetic gases from anaesthetizing locations. Anesthesiology 32(3): 280

V ACCESSORIES TO THE ANAESTHETIC MACHINE AND SPECIAL EQUIPMENT

Lung ventilators

1 Anonymous. 1974. Bennett monitoring spirometer (Hazard). Health Devices 4(2): 50-51

2 Anonymous. 1975. Bennett MA-1 ventilator (Hazards). Health Devices 4 (11/12): 299

3 Anonymous. 1976. Interference with Bourns infant ventilator. Health Devices 5(10): 247

4 Anonymous. 1976. Siemens-Elema servo ventilator 900. Health Devices 6(2): 55

5 Arkinstall, W.W., and Epstein, S.W. 1973. Mechanical failure of a ventilator: A case report. Anesth. Analg. 52(1): 48-52

6 Bethune, D.W., Collis, J.M., and Latimer, R.D. 1976. A safety block for scavenging systems (Apparatus). Anaesthesia 31(9): 1254-1256

7 Bookallil, M.J. 1967. Entrainment of air during mechanical ventilation. Brit. J. Anaesth. 39(2): 184

8 Davies, G., and Tarnawsky, M. 1976. Letter to the Editor. Can. Anaesth. Soc. J. 23(2): 228

9 Desautels, D., and Modell, J.H. 1972. A simple inspiratory safety valve (Clin. Wksp.). Anesthesiology 36(3): 304

10 Dorsch, S.E. 1973. ASA Committee on Mechanical Equipment issues equipment alert. ASA Newsletter 37(11): 8

11 Dunbar, R.W., Redick, L.F., and Merket, T.E. 1970. A safety modification of the Emerson postoperative ventilator (Clin. Wksp.). Anesthesiology 33(5): 555-556

12 Freeman, M.F. 1975. A hazard of the East Radcliffe respirator (Corresp.). Anaesthesia 30(6): 825-826

13 Gamble, J.A.S., and Coppel, D.L. 1973. Potential hazards of expiratory 'retards' in commercial production (Corresp.). Brit. J. Anaesth. 45(5): 533-534

14 Hurdley, J. 1975. A hazard of the East Radcliffe respirator (Corresp.). Anaesthesia 30(6): 825

15 Mayrhofer, O., and Steinbereithner, K. 1967. Some observations on the function of the Bird Mark 8 ventilator (Corresp.). Brit. J. Anaesth. 39(6): 519

16 Mills, M. 1973. Problems with mechanical ventilators. Anesth. Analg. 52(2): 747-752

17 Morrow, D.H., Dixon, W.M., Townley, N.T., and Hebert, C.L. 1965. A safety modification of the air shields ventimeter ventilator (Current Comment). Anesthesiology 26(3): 361-362

18 Overton, J.H., and Miceli, R.M. 1976. A disconnection alarm for the Bennett BA-4 ventilator. Anaesth. Intens. Care 4(2): 159-160

19 Rolbin, S. 1977. An unusual cause of ventilator leak. Can. Anaesth. Soc. J. 24(4): 522-524

20 Sears and Bocar. 1977. Pneumothorax resulting from a closed anesthesia ventilator port (Clin. Reports). Anesthesiology 47(3): 311-313

21 Sia, R.L. 1972. Accidental closure of the expiratory outlet in the Engström ventilator (200) during anaesthesia. A case report. Can. Anaesth. Soc. J. 19(1): 101-104

22 Simionescu, R. 1972. Sticking valve on East-Radcliffe ventilator (Corresp.). Brit. J. Anaesth. 43(11): 1065

23 Spoerel, W.E. The troubles with your anaesthesia machine. Unpublished

24 Turndorf, H., Capan, L., and Kessel, J.W. 1974. Prevention of misconnection of the air-shields ventimeter-ventilator (Brief reports). Anesth. Analg. 53(2): 342-343

25 Waters, D.J. 1968. Factors causing awareness during surgery. Brit. J. Anesth. 40(4): 259-264

26 Wrigley, F.R.H. Letter to the Editor. 1974. Can. Anaesth. Soc. J. 21(4): 434

Humidifiers and nebulizers

1 Anonymous. 1975. Aquatherm aerosol heaters (Hazard). Health Devices 4(6): 222-223

2 Anonymous. 1975. Ohio immersion heaters. Health Devices 5(1): 23

3 Anonymous. 1977. Inspiron disposable nebulizer. Health Devices 6(6): 149-150

4 Dinnick, O.P. Personal communication

5 El-Naggar, M., Collins, V.J., and Francis, H.T. 1973. Fire in an ultrasonic nebulizer (Clin. Wksp.). Anesthesiology 39(3): 339-343

Resuscitators

1 Anonymous. 1974. Life/breather resuscitator (Hazard). Health Devices 3(5): 130-131

2 Maggio, G., and Vogelsanger, G. 1962. Betrachtungen über das Wiederbelebungs- und Narkosegerät für den Aussendienst (Assessment of the apparatus for resuscitation and anaesthesia designed for use outside the hospital). Der Anaesthesist 11(7): 213-217

3 Mathias, J.A. 1968. Neonatal resuscitation (Corresp.). Anaesthesia 23(1): 149

4 Williams, G.F.M., Beasley, W.H., and Fisher, C.B. 1967. The dangers of neonatal resuscitators. Anaesthesia 22(4): 655-658

Hypothermia equipment

1 Anonymous. 1973. Gorman-Rupp Aquamatic-K-Pad (Hazard). Health Devices 2(4): 106

2 Anonymous. 1974. Gaymar hypothermia machine (Hazard). Health Devices 3(9): 229-230
3 Anonymous. 1974. Gorman-Rupp hypothermia unit (Hazard). Health Devices 3(9): 231
4 Anonymous. 1974. Therm-O-Rite hypothermia machine (Hazard). Health Devices 3(9): 232-233

VI EQUIPMENT IN CONTACT WITH THE PATIENT

Airways, masks, nasal catheters, and mouthpieces

1 Ball, C.G., and Berry, F.A. Jr. 1972. A defect in a self-administration anesthesia system (Clin. Wksp.). Anesthesiology 36(5): 509-510
2 Perel, A., Mahler, Y., and Davidson, J.T. 1976. Combustion of a nasal catheter carrying oxygen. Anesthesiology 45(6): 666-667

Tracheal tubes

1 Abramowitz, M.D., and McNabb, T.G. 1976. A new complication of flexo-metallic endotracheal tubes (Corresp.) Brit. J. Anaesth. 48(9): 928
2 Adamson, D.H. 1971. A problem of prolonged oral intubation: case report. Can. Anaesth. Soc. J. 18(2): 213-214
3 Anonymous. 1956. Intubation of the trachea does not absolutely insure a patent airway (Clinical Anesthesia Conference). N.Y. State Med. J. 56(13): 2125-2126
4 Anonymous. 1958. Respiratory obstruction (Clinical Anesthesia Conference). N.Y. State J. Med. 58(10): 1731-1733
5 Anonymous. 1962. Obstruction of the airway in the intubated patient (Clinical Anesthesia Conference). N.Y. State J. Med. 62(1): 83-84
6 Bachand, R., and Fortin, G. 1976. Airway obstruction with cuffed flexo-metallic tracheal tubes. Can. Anaesth. Soc. J. 23(3): 330-333
7 Ballantyne, R.I.W., and Jackson, I. 1954. Anaesthesia for neurosurgical operations. Anaesthesia 9(1): 4-12
8 Bamforth, B.J. 1963. Complications during endotracheal anesthesia. Anesth. Analg. 42(6): 727-733
9 Barnard, J. 1948. An unusual accident during intubation (Corresp.). Anaesthesia 3(3): 126
10 Baron, C.F.J. 1952. Danger from cuffed endotracheal tubes (Corresp.). Brit. Med. J. 2: 391
11 Birkhan, H.J., and Heifetz, M. 1965. 'Uninflatable' inflatable cuffs (Current Comment). Anesthesiology 26(4): 578

12 Blitt, C.D. 1974. Case report: Complete obstruction of an armoured endotracheal tube (Brief Reports). Anesth. Analg. 53(4): 624-625
13 Blott, K. 1954. Endotracheal cuffs (Corresp.). Anaesthesia 9(1): 46
14 Bosomworth, P.P., and Hamelberg, W. 1965. Effect of sterilization techniques on safety and durability of endotracheal tubes and cuffs. Anesth. Analg. 44(5): 576-586
15 Buckley, R.W. 1952. Danger from endotracheal tubes (Corresp.). Brit. Med. J. 2: 939-940
16 Burns, T.H.S. 1956. A danger from flexometallic endotracheal tubes (Corresp.). Brit. Med. J. 1: 439-440
17 Carrie, L.E.S. 1964. A hidden fault in cuffed tubes. Brit. J. Anaesth. 36(1): 58-60
18 Carrington, E. 1976. Ageing of red rubber tubes (Corresp.). Anaesthesia 31(6): 795-796
19 Catane, R., and Davidson, J.T. 1969. A hazard of cuffed flexo-metallic endotracheal tubes. Brit. J. Anaesth. 41(12): 1086
20 Child, D.A., and Ali, M.M. 1977. A hazard of the Pollard endotracheal tube. Brit. J. Anaesth. 49(2): 179-181
21 Chiu, T.M., and Meyers, E.F. 1976. Defective disposable endotracheal tube (Brief Reports). Anesth. Analg. 55(3): 437
22 Clarke, A.D. 1962. The White double lumen tube: A report on its use in 50 cases. Brit. J. Anaesth. 34(11): 822-824
23 Clark, M.M. 1964. 'Put not your trust in tubes.' Brit. J. Anaesth. 36(8): 519-520
24 Clausen, J.R. 1949. An unusual accident during intubation (Corresp.). Anaesthesia 4(2): 45
25 Cohen, D.D., and Dillon, J.B. 1972. Hazards of armoured endotracheal tubes. Anesth. Analg. 51(6): 856-858
26 Cohen, P.J. 1977. An endotracheal-tube barb (Corresp.). Anesthesiology 47(1): 77
27 Davies, A., and Rowlands, D.E. 1971. Endotracheal tubes (Clinical Forum). Anaesthesia 26(1): 79
28 Davies, R.M. 1963. Faulty construction of a re-inforced latex endotracheal tube. Brit. J. Anaesth. 35(2): 128-130
29 Debnath, S.K., and Waters, D.J. 1968. Leaking cuffed endotracheal tubes two case reports (Corresp.). Brit. J. Anaesth. 40(10): 807
30 Divekar, V.M. 1967. Rupture of a cuffed tube (Corresp.). Anaesthesia 22(3): 531
31 Doane, W.A. 1956. Occlusion of endotracheal tube by overinflated cuff (Clinical Anesthesia Conference). N.Y. State J. Med. 56(24): 3936-3937

32 Doyle, L.A., and Conway, C.F. 1967. A hazard of cuffed endotracheal tubes (Case Report). Anaesthesia 22(1): 140-141

33 Dryden, G.E. 1977. Circulatory collapse after pneumonectomy (an unusual complication from the use of a Carlens catheter). Case Report. Anesth. Analg. 56(3): 451-452

34 Dunn, G.L. 1975. Letter to the Editor. Can. Anaesth. Soc. J. 22(3): 379-380

35 Dutton, C.S. 1962. A bizarre case of obstruction in an Oxford non-kink endotracheal tube (Corresp.). Anaesthesia 17(3): 395-396

36 Edwards, G., Morton, H.J.V., Pask, E.A., and Wylie, W.D. 1956. Deaths associated with anaesthesia: A report of 1000 cases. Anaesthesia 11(3): 194-220

37 Elliott, C.J.R. 1973. Problems of cuff deflation (Apparatus). Anaesthesia 28(5): 535-537

38 Forrester, A.C. 1959. Mishaps in anaesthesia. Anaesthesia 14(4): 388-399

39 Franklin, C.B. 1973. Robertshaw endo-bronchial tubes. Variation in specification or production (Corresp.). Anaesthesia 28(3): 343

40 Gilston, A. 1969. Obstruction of endotracheal tube (Case Report). Anaesthesia 24(2): 256

41 Gold, M.I., and Atwood, J.M. 1965. Respiratory obstruction (Case Reports). Anesthesiology 26(4): 577-578

42 Gosepath, J., Puente-Egido, J.J., and Ischokl-Heinrichs, H. 1967. Zwischenfall während Endotrachealer Intubation (Accident during endotracheal intubation). Der Anaesthesist 16(4): 112-113

43 Gould, A.B., and Seldon, T.H. 1968. An unusual complication with a cuffed endotracheal tube. Anesth. Analg. 47(3): 239-240

44 Hale Enderby, G.E. 1961. Tapered nylon-reinforced latex endotracheal tubes (New Inventions). Lancet II (7204): 693

45 Hale Enderby, G.E. 1977. Tapered nylon-reinforced latex endotracheal tubes (Corresp.). Anaesthesia 32(9): 920-921

46 Haselhuhn, D.H. 1958. Case report — Occlusion of endotracheal tube with foreign body. Anesthesiology 19(4): 561-562

47 Hayes, B. 1961. Respiratory obstruction due to faulty Carlens endotracheal tube (Corresp.). Lancet 2: 1205-1206

48 Hedden, M., Smith, R.B.F., and Torpey, D.J. 1972. A complication of metal spiral-imbedded latex endotracheal tubes. Anesth. Analg. 51(6): 859-862

49 Hoffman, S., and Freedman, M. 1976. Delayed lumen obstruction in endotracheal tubes. Brit. J. Anaesth 48(10): 1025-1028

50 Hogarth, B. 1976. Ageing of red rubber tubes (Corresp.). Anaesthesia 31(6): 795

51 Holland, R. 1970. R. Australasian College of Surgeons Seminar: 'Safety in Operating Theatres.' Melbourne (Quoted by Dinnick)

52 Hudson, M.C., and Ross, A.W. 1973. An unusual defect in a Robertshaw tube (Corresp.). Anaesthesia 28(3): 344-345

53 Jacobson, J. 1969. A hazard of armoured endotracheal anesthesia. Anesth. Analg. 48(1): 37-41

54 Jenkins, A.V. 1959. Unexpected hazard of anaesthesia (Corresp.). Lancet 1: 761-762

55 Jenkins, V. 1963. Unusual difficulty with double-lumen endo-bronchial tube (Corresp.). Anaesthesia 18(2): 236-237

56 Kamen, J.M., and Wilkinson, C. 1977. Removal of an inflated endotracheal tube cuff (Corresp.). Anesthesiology 46(4): 308-309

57 Ketover, A.K., and Feingold, A. 1975. Collapse of a disposable endotracheal tube by its high pressure cuff (Clin. Reports). Anesthesiology 43(1): 108-110

58 Kleine, J.W., and Moesker, A. 1972. Endotracheal tubes (Corresp.). Anaesthesia 27(1): 104-105

59 Koch, H., and Franke, I. 1973. Eine neue Komplikation der endotrachealen Intubation (A new complication of endotracheal intubation) (Fehler und Gefahren) Der Anaesthesist 22(10): 466-467

60 Kohli, M.S., and Manku, R.S. 1966. Reinforced endotracheal tube. Diversion of air from cuff balloon causing obstruction. Anesthesiology 27(4): 513-514

61 Lewis, R.N., and Swerdlow, M. 1964. Hazards of endotracheal intubation. Brit. J. Anaesth. 36(8): 504-515

62 Liew, R.P.C. 1975. Respiratory obstruction with an Oxford tube (Corresp.). Anaesthesia 30(4): 558-559

63 Linder, G.S. 1974. A new polyolefin-coated endotracheal tube stylet. Anesth. Analg. 53(2): 341-342

64 MacIntosh, R.R. 1949. Deaths under anaesthetics. Brit. J. Anaesth. 21(3): 107-136

65 Malone, B.T. 1975. A complication of Rusch armoured endotracheal tubes. Anesth. Analg. 54(6): 756

66 Marshall, J. 1968. Self-lubricated stylet for endotracheal tubes. Anesthesiology 29(2): 385

67 Mimpriss, T.J. 1972. Respiratory obstruction due to a round worm (Corresp.). Brit. J. Anaesth. 44(4): 413

68 Mirakhur, R.K. 1974. Airway obstruction with cuffed armoured tracheal tubes. Can. Anaesth. Soc. J. 21(2): 251-253

69 Ng, T.Y., and Datta, T.D. 1976. Difficult extubation of an endotracheal tube cuff (Brief Reports). Anesth. Analg. 55(6): 876-877

70 Ng, T.Y., and Kirimli, B.I. 1975. Hazards in use of anode endotracheal tube: A case report and review. Anesth. Analg. 54(6): 710-714

71 Pavlin, E.G., Van Nimwegan, D., and Hornbein, T.F. 1975. Failure of a high-compliance low-pressure cuff to prevent aspiration (Clin. Reports). Anesthesiology 42(2): 216-219

72 Peers, B. 1975. Foreign bodies in endotracheal tubes (Corresp.). Anaesth. Intens. Care 3(3): 267

73 Pelagio, Layug, Wilder, R., and Safar, P. 1959. Airway obstruction during pneumonectomy (Case Report). Anesthesiology 20(3): 385-386

74 Perel, A., Katzenelson, R., Klein, E. and Cotev, S. 1977. Collapse of endotracheal tubes due to overinflation of high-compliance cuffs (Clin. Reports). Anesth. Analg. 56(5): 731-733

75 Phillips, B. 1971. Defect in a cuffed tube (Clinical Forum). Anaesthesia 26(2): 237

76 Pollard, B. 1977. The Pollard endotracheal tube (Corresp.). Brit. J. Anaesth. 49(10): 1069-1070

77 Powell, D. Russel. 1974. Obstruction to endotracheal tubes (Corresp.). Brit. J. Anaesth. 46(4): 252

78 Price, J. Middleton. 1952. Danger from endotracheal tubes (Corresp.). Brit. Med. J. 2: 939

79 Pryer, D.L., Pryer, R.D., and Williams, A.F. 1960. Fatal respiratory obstruction due to faulty endotracheal tube (Corresp.). Lancet 2: 742-743

80 Robbie, D.S., and Pearce, D.J. 1959. Some dangers of armoured tubes. Anaesthesia 14(4): 379-385

81 Robertshaw, F.L. 1973. Robertshaw endo-bronchial tubes. A reply (Corresp.). Anesthesia 28(3): 344

82 Roland, P., and Stovner, J. 1975. Brain damage following collapse of a polyvinyl tube: Elasticity and rermeability of the cuff. Acta Anaesth. Scandin. 19(4): 303-309

83 Rollason, W.N. 1952. Danger from endotracheal tubes (Corresp.). Brit. Med. J. 2: 616

84 Salt, R.H. 1976. Respiratory obstruction with an Oxford tube (Corresp.). Anaesthesia 31(1): 108-109

85 Scheinfelder, A. 1973. Misadventure during endotracheal anaesthesia (Corresp.). JAMA 225(5): 524

86 Schmidt, W. 1971. Über eine seltene Komplikation bei Versuch der Extubation (A rare complication of extubation) (Fehler und Gefahren). Der Anaesthesist 20(5): 195

87 Seuffert, G.W., and Urbach, K.F. 1958. An additional hazard of endotracheal intubation. Can. Anaesth. Soc. J. 15(3): 300-301

88 Smotrina, M.M., Nagel, E.C., and Moya, F. 1966. Failure of inflatable cuff resulting in foreign body in the Trachea. Anesthesiology 27(4): 512

89 Sobel, A.M. 1964. Obstructed endotracheal catheter (Current Comment). Anesthesiology 25(4): 581

90 Stanley, T.H. 1974. Effects of anesthetic gases on endotracheal tube cuff gas volumes (Brief Reports). Anesth. Analg. 53(3): 480-482

91 Stanley, T.H. 1975. Nitrous oxide and the pressures and volumes of high- and low-pressure endotracheal tube cuffs in intubated patients. Anesthesiology 42(5): 637-640

92 Stanley, T.H., Foote, J.L., and Liu, W.S. 1975. A simple pressure relief valve to prevent increases in endotracheal tube cuff pressure and volume in intubated patients (Clin. Reports). Anesthesiology 43(4): 478-481

93 Stark, D.C.C., and Pask, E.A. 1962. Central sterile supply of endotracheal tubes. The effect of autoclaving on the life of mineral rubber endotracheal tubes. Anaesthesia 17(2): 195-207

94 Tahir, A.H., and Adriani, J. 1971. Failure to effect satisfactory seal after hyperinflation of endotracheal cuff. Anesth. Analg. 50(4): 540-543

95 Tavacoli, M., and Corssen, G. 1976. An unusual case of difficult extubation (Clin. Reports). Anesthesiology 45(5): 552-553

96 Tofany, V.J. 1961. Occlusion of endotracheal catheter (Case Report). Anesthesiology 22(1): 124-125

97 Walton, F.A. 1967. Obstruction of the lumen of new endotracheal tubes. Can. Anaesth. Soc. J. 14(6): 605-606

98 Walton, W.J. 1967. An invaginated tube (Corresp.). Brit. J. Anaesth. 39(6): 520

99 Waters, R.M., and Gillespie, N.A. 1944. Deaths in the operating room. Anesthesiology 5(2): 113-128

100 Wong, R.M. 1977. Case report: Complication of a polyvinyl chloride endotracheal tube. Anaesth. Intens. Care 5(1): 78-79

101 Wong, R.M. 1977. An unusual source of leakage from the cuff of a tracheal tube. (Corresp.). Anaesth. Intens. Care 5(4): 389

102 Yeung, M.L., and Lett, Z. 1974. An uncommon hazard of armoured endotracheal tubes (Apparatus). Anaesthesia 29(2): 186-187

103 Zeitlin, G.L., Short, D.H., and Ryder, G.H. 1965. An assessment of the Robertshaw double-lumen tube. Brit. J. Anaesth. 37(11): 858-860

Tracheostomy tubes

1 Berkebile, P.E., and Smith, R. Brian. 1972. Pre-stretched cuffs on tracheostomy tubes (Corresp.). Brit. J. Anaesth. 45(2): 234

2 Chamney, A.R. 1969. Humidification requirements and techniques.
Including a review of the performance of equipment in current use. Anaesthesia 24(4): 602-617
3 Holdcroft, A., Loh, L., and Lumley, J. 1974. Acceptability of swivel connectors. Brit. J. Anaesth. 46(4): 298-301
4 Holdcroft, A., and Lumley, J. 1975. Swivel connections (Corresp.). Brit.
J. Anaesth. 47(5): 642-643
5 Kosik, G. and Todor, G. 1968. 'Cuff-Aneurysma' bei Trachealkanülen
(Aneurysm of the cuff in tracheostomy tubes). Der Anaesthesist 17(7):
235-236
6 Lawson, D.R. 1973. Pre-stretched cuffs on tracheostomy tubes (Corresp.).
Brit. J. Anaesth. 45(2): 234
7 Pavlin, E.G., Nelson, E., and Pulliam, J. 1976. Difficulty in removal of
tracheostomy tubes (Clin. Reports). Anesthesiology 44(1): 69-70
8 Röse, W. 1963. Verlegung einer Trachealkanüle durch einen aspirierten Zahn
(Obstruction of a tracheostomy tube by an inhaled tooth) (Fehler und
Gefahren). Der Anaesthesist 12(10): 319
9 Wandless, J.G., Emery, F.M., Evans, J., and Foley, R.J.E. 1972. Pre-stretched
cuffs on tracheostomy tubes (Corresp.). Brit. J. Anaesth. 44(11): 1222
10 Ware, J.R. 1975. A hazard of Portex soft seal tracheostomy tubes with
swivel connectors (Corresp.). Brit. J. Anaesth. 47(12): 1339

Magill forceps and laryngeal sprays

1 Beer, E.G. 1949. Breakage of a Magill forcep. A case report. Anesthesiology
10(4): 511-512
2 Dinnick, O.P. Personal communication
3 Evers, H. 1973. A hazard due to a commercially available topical spray
(Corresp.). Anaesthesia 28(6): 709
4 Francis, J.G. 1967. A wandering spray nozzle. Brit. J. Anaesth. 39(10):
813-814
5 Liew, P.C. 1973. A hazard due to a commercially available topical spray
(Corresp.). Anaesthesia 28(3): 346
6 Paymaster, N.J. 1972. A serious potential hazard of the MacIntosh
laryngeal spray (Corresp.). Brit. J. Anaesth. 44(12): 1333

Needles for injection

1 Ballie, N.M., and Catton, D.V. 1975. Letter to the Editor. Can. Anaesth.
Soc. J. 22(4): 529

2 Bonica, J.J. 1953. *The Management of Pain.* Lea and Febiger, Philadelphia, pp. 216, 223

3 Bonica, J.J. 1967. *Principles and Practice of Obstetric Analgesia and Anesthesia.* F.A. Davis Company, Philadelphia, pp. 483, 608

4 Charlebois, P.A. 1966. Coring: The unseen menace. Can. Anaesth. Soc. J. 13(6): 585-597

5 Crawford Little, D. 1955. Skin fragments in end-opening needles (Clin. and Lab. Notes). Can. Med. Assoc. J. 72(5): 374-375

6 Eng, M., and Zorotovich, R.A. 1977. Broken-needle complication with a disposable introducer. Anesthesiology 46(2): 147-148

7 Gibson, T., and Norris, W. 1958. Skin fragments removed by injection needles. Lancet II (7054): 983-985

8 Magath, T.B., and McLellan, J.T. 1950. Reaction to accidentally injected rubber plugs. Am. J. Clin. Path. 20(9): 829-833

9 Moore, D.C. 1955. *Complications of Regional Anaesthesia.* Charles C. Thomas, Springfield, Ill. pp. 243-245

10 Moore, D.C. 1955. *Regional Block*, 4th ed. Charles C. Thomas, Springfield, Ill. pp. 50, 256

11 Odom, N.J., and Heath, M.L. 1977. A dangerous disposable epidural needle. Anaesthesia 32(1): 75

12 Snow, J.C., Kripke, B.J., Sakellarides, H., and Patel, K.P. 1974. Broken disposable needle during an axillary approach to block the brachial plexus. Anesth. Analg. 53(1): 89-92

Intravenous cannulae and catheters

1 Al-Abrak, M.H. and Samuel, J.R. 1974. An unusual cause of breaking of a central venous catheter (Case Report). Anaesthesia 29(5): 585-587

2 Anonymous. 1977. Latex balloons on wedge-pressure catheters. Health devices 6(5): 123-124

3 Beaulieu, M., and Gravel, J.A. 1961. Cardiotomie pour ablation d'un catheter intraveineux. Laval Med. 31(4): 458-461

4 Brown, C.A., and Kent, A. 1956. Perforation of right ventricle by polyethylene catheter lost during intravenous therapy. Sout. Med. J. 49(5): 466-467

5 Colvin, M.P., Savege, T.M., and Lewis, C.T. 1975. Pulmonary damage from a Swan-Ganz catheter (Case Report). Brit. Anaesth. 47(10): 1107-1109

6 Cook, T.L., and Duecker, W. 1976. Tension pneumothorax following internal jugular cannulation. Anesthesiology 45(5): 554-555

7 Coppel, D.L., and Samuel, I.O. 1974. A complication of long venous catheters (Case Report). Anaesthesia 29(2): 175-177

8 Doering, R.B., Stemmer, E.A., and Connolly, J.E. 1967. Complications of indwelling venous catheters. With particular reference to catheter embolus. 1967. Am. J. Surg. 114(2): 259-266

9 Gooding, J.M., and Tavakoli, M. 1977. Inability to remove the metal stylet from a central venous catheter (Corresp.). Brit. J. Anaesth. 49(4): 396

10 Hammermeister, K.E., and Kennedy, J.W. 1968. Removal of broken cardiac catheters (Corresp.). New Engl. J. Med. 278(16): 911

11 Harken, Lt. Col. D.E., and Zoll, Major P.M. 1946. Foreign bodies in and in relation to the thoracic blood vessels and heart. Am. Heart J. 32(1): 1-19

12 Henley, F.T., and Ballard, J.W. 1969. Percutaneous removal of flexible foreign body from the heart (Technical Notes). Radiology 92(1): 176

13 Juhl, B. 1973. Percutaneous removal of a catheter-embolism from the right side of the heart. A case report. Acta Anaesth. Scandin. 17(1): 37-40

14 Kux, M., and Kutscha-Lissberg, E. 1968. Die Gefahr der Katheterembolie beim oberen Hohlen-Venenkatheter (Danger of catheter embolus from superior vena cava catheters). Der Anaesthesist, 17(7): 232-234

15 Lipp, H., O'Donoghue, K., and Resnekov, L. 1971. Intracardiac knotting of a flow-directed balloon catheter. New Engl. J. Med. 284(4): 220

16 Massumi, R.A., and Ross, A.M. 1967. Atraumatic, non-surgical technique for removal of broken catheters from cardiac cavities. New Engl. J. Med. 277(4): 195-196

17 McNabb, T.G., Green, L.H., and Parker, F.L. 1975. A potentially serious complication with Swan-Ganz catheter placement by the percutaneous jugular route. Brit. J. Anaesth. 47(8): 895-897

18 Miller, R.E., Cockerill, E.M., and Helbig, H. 1970. Percutaneous removal of catheter emboli from the pulmonary arteries. Radiology 94(1): 151-153

19 Moncrief, Lt. Col. J.A. Femoral catheters. Ann. Surg. 147(2): 166-172

20 Ranniger, K. 1968. An instrument for retrieval of intravascular foreign bodies. Radiology 91(5): 1043-1044

21 Schechter, E., and Parisi, A. 1972. Removal of catheter fragments from pulmonary artery using a snare. Brit. Heart J. 34(7): 699-700

22 Schwartz, A.J. 1977. Percutaneous aortic catheterization − A hazard of supraclavicular internal-jugular-vein catheterization. Anesthesiology 46(1): 77

23 Shin, B., McAslan, T.C., and Ayella, R.J. 1975. Problems with measurements using the Swan-Ganz catheter (Clin. Reports). Anesthesiology 43(4): 474-476

24 Smyth, N.P.D., Boivin, M.R., and Bacos, J.M. 1968. Transjugular removal of foreign body from right atrium by endoscopic forceps. J. Thorac. Cardiovasc. Surg. 55(4): 594-597

25 Swan, H.J.C. 1968. *Complications related to equipment failure. Cooperative Study on Cardiac Catheterization* (Monograph No. 20). Ed. E. Braunwald and H.J.C. Swan. Am. Heart Assoc., New York, pp. 57-58

26 Swaroop, S. 1972. Knotting of two central venous monitoring catheters. Am. J. Med. 53(3): 386-388

27 Talmage, E.A. 1976. Shearing hazard of intra-arterial teflon catheters (Brief Reports). Anesth. Analg. 55(4): 597-598

28 Taylor, F.W., and Rutherford, C.E. 1963. Accidental loss of plastic tube into venous system. Arch. Surg. 86(2): 177-179

29 Trusler, G.A., and Mustard, W.T. 1958. Intravenous polyethylene catheter successfully removed from the heart (Case Report). Can. Med. Assoc. J. 79(7): 558-559

30 Turner, D.D., and Sommers, S.C. 1954. Accidental passage of a polyethlene catheter from cubital vein to right atrium. Report of a fatal case (Med. Intell.). New Engl. J. Med. 251(18): 744-745

31 Van Dijk, B., and Bakker, P.M. 1977. Appraisal of the dislocation of central venous catheter tips using subclavian and arm veins. Der Anaesthesist 26(3): 138-140

32 Wellmann, K.F., Reinhard, A., and Salazar, E.P. 1968. Polyethylene catheter embolism. Review of the literature and report of a case with associated fatal tricuspid and systemic candidiasis. Circulation 37(3): 380-392

Epidural catheters

1 Abouleish, E. 1974. Preventing and detecting leakage in epidural catheters (Brief Reports). Anesth. Analg. 53(3): 474-475

Index